Praise for *Keep Looking Up...*

"When I think back on seeing Kim during her battle with cancer, I just remember how cute and stylish she looked in her bandana; she made cancer almost look cool. Positive was an understatement and all the while she was taking care of a good friend who was battling cancer who succumbed to her illness. I could only hope to handle an illness with such grace, but hope I never have to."

-Anne Lehotsky,
friend and former co-worker

"I've known Kim for at least 15 years and I've never known her to despair. She is courageous in facing life, especially when it gets tough. She is a busy working wife who still makes time to visit and to help others. She was most kind to my family during the time of my beloved wife's passing due to ovarian cancer. Thank you for the kindness you have shown us, Kim."

-Hank Whitmore,
former Presbyterian Elder and retired airline pilot

"I have known Kim since her second visit to Florida Cancer Specialists on May 14, 2008. From that day and even today, three years later, every time she comes through the office door, she lights up the office. She has a hopeful and cheerful presence all the time. I was excited for the patients in the chemo room when Kim was coming in. I knew the day would be fun and exciting—especially with her bouquet of balloons she would bring in. Kim faced a very difficult situation with a positive outlook and she is a success. I know in my heart many people benefited from this as well."

-Beth Jensen
front staff, check in desk
Florida Cancer Specialists

More Praise for **_Keep Looking Up..._**

"I have known Kim for six years, and she is a remarkable woman. Her faith is certainly what has led her to this point in her life. She has always had a very positive attitude. I wish I could be more like Kim!"

-Gretchen VanKula,
friend and former co-worker

"Thank you for thinking of Lori while writing your book. Nothing can replace Lori, but her memory lives on in words and deeds. When I feel sad and lonely I always pick up the box of kisses you presented to me. It was such a memorable and moving gift. I am always filled with the spirit of joy and happiness. Thank you again."

-*Your friend always,* Bill

"How could I ever forget the first day Kim walked, or rather "sailed" into our treatment room. Here was this very tiny person, dressed to the nines with this GIANT Cher wig on! Without the wig, she was maybe five feet, with the wig, maybe six. "So, why the Cher lookalike?" I asked. Kim tells me, "I wanted to know how it would be without hair." Now, she has these big round eyes that look right at you, and you have to speak truthfully.

"With your attitude, you are going to do well," I tell her. And she did. She always arrived with a fanfare, giving out sandwiches and candy and balloons to the other patients, talking the whole time she was receiving treatment. I tried to tell her new jokes each time she came, and she gave me jokes right back. Kim was and is, an inspiration to both staff and patients. It may sound strange to hear, but I'm glad she was a part of my professional career as a chemotherphy pharmacy tech. Keep the faith, baby!"

-Jerry Pulliam, CPht,
Florida Cancer Specialists

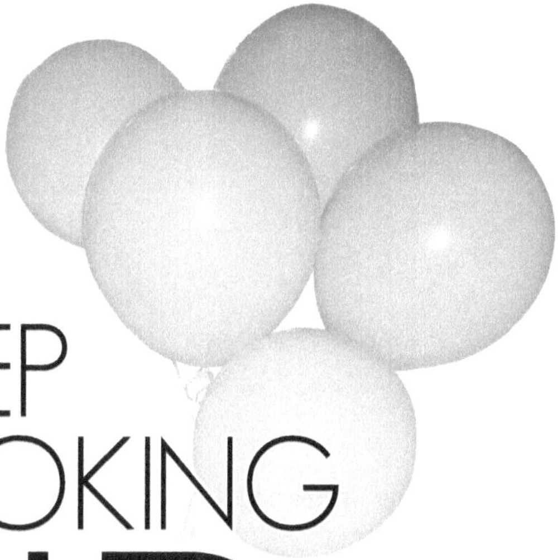

KEEP LOOKING UP

Kim McAuliffe Clark

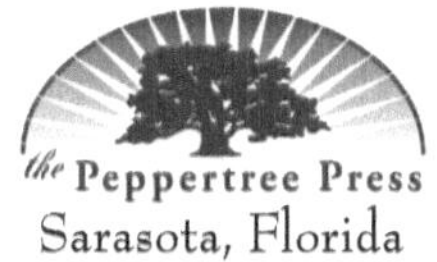

the Peppertree Press
Sarasota, Florida

For information regarding permission,
call 941-922-2662 or contact us at our website:
www.peppertreepublishing.com or write to:
the Peppertree Press, LLC.
Attention: Publisher
1269 First Street, Suite 7
Sarasota, Florida 34236

ISBN: 978-1-936343-64-5

Library of Congress Number: 2011920733

Printed in the U.S.A.

Printed February 2011

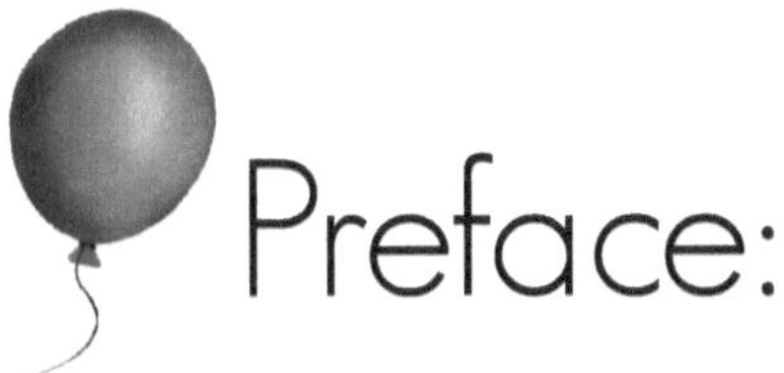# Preface:

If you are going through difficulties,

then you came to the right place.

You are looking for answers

and God lead you to this book,

there must be a message here for you.

I hope that you find peace.

Dedication

I am so thankful to be able to dedicate this book to the Lord. He leads me. He has truly blessed me in so many ways. "Thank you Lord."

If it is His will, I would like the opportunity to write another book or two.

Honorable Mentions:

Thank you Tim Clark, my wonderful husband of 14 years. And to

Heather Rae and Michele Bea (our two beautiful and talented girls) for being so loving, giving and strong during the trying times. I love you all so much.

To my precious mom and dad, (David and Cecelia McAuliffe) thank you for all your help, support and endless love – you are the best friends a daughter could ever have, I love you both dearly.

To David McAuliffe, my brother, I love you pal.

To Ray and Ferne Clark and to the Leath Family, Chris, Kelly, Kendall and Matthew.

Home away from home. Alabama is so much sweeter thanks to all of you. Roll Tide!

To Michele DelMonaco, my fine Italian friend of 24 years. You have been like a sister to me and I love you as one.

To Phyllis Siskel, I will never forget all of your encouragement. Blessings my dear friend and thank you.

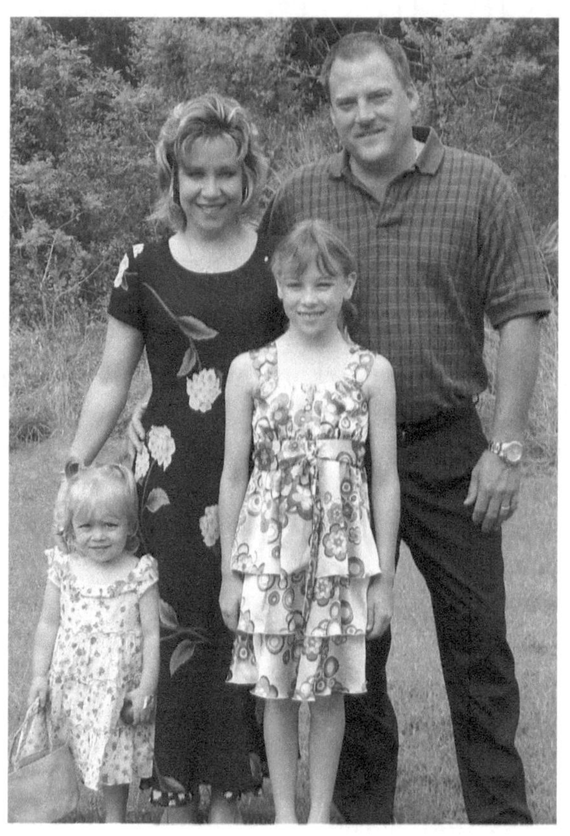

Meet the Clark's. I'm Kim, my husband Tim & our two girls, Heather (at age 10) and Michele (at age 2). This was taken Easter Sunday, March 23, 2008.

See, I had the same hairstyle for about 17 years (long, blonde & curly) and just prior to this I had a sudden urge to change my look. Now that I've been through what I've been through, I feel thas sudden urge to change my look was yet another way that God prepared me for what was yet to come.

CHAPTER 1

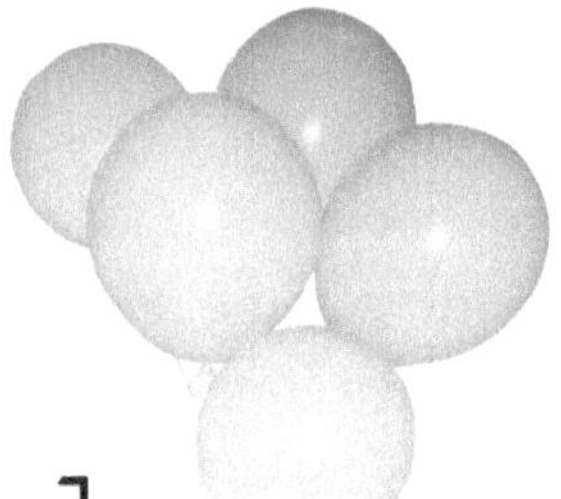

A lady noticed I was crying today she softly tapped me on the shoulder and said, "Better things are yet to come." It was my message. This morning I specifically asked the Lord to please send me "a sign." When I prayed I said, "Lord, I just don't know what you want me to do or where you want me to be, so please send me a sign, but please make it obvious." I don't always notice the subtle.

I'm in the middle of an emotional funk. Should I look for a job? Should I just stay home? I'm bitter being in this situation to begin with. Being laid off from a job that I absolutely loved, which I was totally committed to for the past five years has been one of the biggest obstacles for me. I just can't seem to shake the despair and sadness of it. The loss of half of our income has brought me stress and emotional frustration that

I can't even explain. Immediately, we stopped going out, stopped shopping, we do without – including some necessities! With these mandatory changes comes depression and even some anger.

My family and I have certainly had our share of trials over the last 12 years. I've learned that Christians do. Christians are going to go through more tests and more trials, and as we ask for the Lord's help, we will overcome them. Maybe not in the time frame we would like, but we will overcome them.

I'm not some "holy roller," but I have been a Christian since the age of 10. I'm still human and I'm still a sinner. I've been a sinning human every day of my life. This means I have good days, bad days, great days and very bad days just like everyone else. I have made poor choices and bad decisions. I don't always use the best language, and I'm working hard on that. The good news about being a Christian is, I can seek forgiveness, I can seek God's help with anything, and by my faith I know He will not forsake me. I am blessed. I may not have a job, but I'm still blessed.

I've been through some tough things and I want everyone to know, if God can bring me through these things, he can bring you through your challenges too. Just give your troubles over to God – let Him handle it. That's what I did.

I'll do my best to tell you what I've been through and how God lead me through.

When I was living in North Carolina, I look back at how lonely I was. I had been single almost five years at that time. I remember asking God why I wasn't in a loving relationship. Why not me?

Initially, I had moved to North Carolina in 1989 with an individual I should have never been involved with. I was young (22) and determined. I made a commitment and I was going to stick it out and make it work. We were together almost three years and we were now moving to North Carolina. I was heartbroken about leaving my family and Florida.

After many prayers, many many months of sadness, mental abuse and living with someone who constantly belittled me and who hated life, I left him the following year.

My family in Florida had their share of troubles as my parents and grandparents were together in the car and had an accident. My grandmother broke her toe, my mom broke her foot, and my dad hit the wind shield with his head and had a concussion and my grandfather, the driver....I don't believe he was injured.

My mom, who works as a hair dresser, had

pretty painful injuries and had to have surgery on her foot. Recovery wouldn't be quick and it wasn't. With injuries come pretty hefty bills and with that, setbacks. This was one of those times.

I knew my family wasn't in a good physical or financial place. All I wanted them to know was I was healthy, single and able to take care of myself. I had goals of saving and moving back to Florida and I hoped and prayed they wouldn't worry about me. The fact was I was absolutely broke even though I had four jobs (I worked full-time at Baker Furniture as an Engineering Clerk, Part-time at Ingles Super Market, as a cashier, I waitressed nights at Rick's Restaurant and I also waitressed weekends at Puccio's Family Restaurant). I had wonderful friends in North Carolina....but I had goals of moving back home as soon as I could.

I learned a lot living alone and learned a lot about myself. I wasn't the partying type whatso-ever. I wasn't big on drinking, although I drank socially and back then I smoked cigarettes a little. Most of my North Carolina friends would say, "You don't need to drink to be fun little Kim you're too much fun already." I'm proud to say, most of the time when I went out with my friends, I was the designated driver! There were times I felt I was only invited for that very purpose, but I didn't mind. I needed to keep my head and wanted to be sure to take care of me. I get that from my dad. Be aware of your surroundings, keep your head up & stay alert. I couldn't do that if I was flopping all over the place drunk.

My close friends know I am a proud and able gun owner. I'm slightly paranoid and over cautious. I also get that from my dad, but I was even more cautious living there (North Carolina).

I continued to live the next four years alone in Andrews, North Carolina. The town absolutely adopted me as their own. Kind, warm, loving people surrounded me; I was never alone for a holiday or special occasion I was always thought of by someone where I lived or where I worked. I would be asked over to their homes frequently.

Thank you for the kindnesses and your friendship – Carol Gibson, Cheryl Lovingood, April Sherrill, Tommy Messer, Rhonda Smiley, Patty Puccio, Larry "Goat" Daily, and Tom Hurley.

I went on dates here and there but nothing serious. I just didn't seem to get involved with anyone long term. There was one guy, I dated for a couple of years, but it wasn't exclusive and he lived three hours away.

Testimony—A transmission from God

So, this one day I began planning my first solo visit to Florida. There was a four-day weekend/ holiday coming up, plus I had a couple vacation days. It would be a perfect time to visit my family, but I wanted it to be a surprise visit. I began checking in with the family often, making sure they would be in town. My parents even asked if there was a way I could make a trip – but I assured them I would be fine and I really didn't want to use up my precious vacation days. I was so excited planning this, just showing up from North Carolina. I would giggle with excitement just thinking about it. I planned this for at least two months, counting my pennies, making sure the bills were paid and I had enough for gas there and back again, it would be close, but it could be done. Each day I would count down the days to my trip. I would be in Florida in one week. As I daydreamed about my trip, I got into the car on my way to work and the car doesn't start. I'm thinking, "What now?" I got the car over to Tommy (my co-worker and dear friend April's dad who is a preacher and a mechanic) yes, he's an honest mechanic indeed. Tommy calls later with the diagnosis. Although I didn't worry about getting around town, with all my friends to help out....but, there wasn't much of a chance of taking a trip to Florida without a transmission! When I asked him what kind of cost was involved with something like this....less labor it was something like $850-900 for a new transmission and $350-400 for a rebuilt one, with no guarantee!! I was positively crushed. There was no way I could afford to fix the car before this trip. I was so sad. I was in a state of total despair and depression and I couldn't tell my family because it was supposed to be a surprise. I didn't feel like eating, working or socializing, nothing. I just sat and cried. It had been nearly three years since I saw my family and just when I'm planning to see them a disaster happens. Why? Wasn't I entitled to see them? I was in that miserable relationship for four years, alone in North Carolina another four years, hadn't seen my family in almost three, and everyone else had a boyfriend except for me. Why was all of this happening?

I remember going to work the next day, so depressed. April was so kind to let me borrow a vehicle for as long as I needed. I immediately left work. I had to clear my head. I wanted to ask God what He wanted. He obviously was trying to get my attention. I thought of driving to some isolated spot to pray, but I think I needed to "face Him." But how? I drove around town and figured I should drive to church, but what church? I hadn't attended any churches in North Carolina. I was Presbyterian and every church in town seemed to be Baptist. I thought I remembered a little Presbyterian church just off the main street; I decided to stop by to see if the pastor is in. I walked into this little church it was dark and quiet it reminded me of the school house/church on Little House on the Prairie. The wooden floor creaked and the building was old. I called out, "Hello?" and heard the creaking of a chair in the back where a little light was on. Out walked Pastor Hamilton with a big smile and cheerful "hello." I was on the verge of crying. I needed to tell this man how upset I was. I suppose the expression on my face was all the guidance Pastor Hamilton needed. I told him I was going through a difficult time and I think there was a purpose that I wound up here. Almost without introductions I got started on my tangent. I instantly started to cry. I told the pastor who I was, how long I lived in that town, how unhappy I had been living alone all these years, I hadn't seen my family in nearly three years and just as I was planning a surprise trip, my vehicle takes a dump on me. I asked the pastor why God needed my attention and if he would let God know I'm here to do whatever He needs, but why won't God allow me to visit my family? After spilling my troubles and going through a box of tissues, this kind and attentive Pastor offered to pray with me and He prayed for me.

We talked for a very long time and learned a little bit about each other. He asked me where I worked, where I lived and about my family in Florida. We talked about many things that will come up later on in the book, but just as I was about to go back to work, the pastor asked me to look him in the eye and answer a question. He said, "Do you believe that you will see your family next weekend?" With curiosity, I replied "Well, I want to but it doesn't look like..." He repeated his question, "Do you believe you will see your family next weekend?" I hesitated but replied "Yes." He smiled and said, "Good, now go back to work and have a better day." I thanked him, but now I was wondering what kind of conversation I just had. I left there feeling so much better, relieved but with a twist. I'm going to FL? But how? My car is in the shop, I don't have a dime to get it fixed and I'm supposed to pack for a trip? When I got to work, I told April about the conversation I had with Pastor Hamilton. Her dad still had my vehicle. I told her I didn't have the money to pay him, so I couldn't authorize him to work on it.

I kept myself busy by working and didn't let

myself worry about the car or the trip. I carried on as if the car wasn't broken. I was so thankful that April allowed me to use her spare vehicle to get around town.

Friday morning before I was to get on the road to Florida, Tommy called me to tell me my car should be fixed by Saturday morning. At first I couldn't believe my ears. It was almost fixed. I was so excited, then petrified with fear, thinking, "How was I going to pay for this?" I never asked him to fix it. All I could say was "Ok? That sounds great. What should I do?" He said I should just hope the part is delivered today so that he can put it in and test it out. I thought of asking questions, but didn't because Pastor Hamilton said all I was to do was to believe and pack for FL.

The next morning I had two stuffed bags, was eating breakfast and sipping on coffee when Tommy pulled up in my car. I can't even bring to words the feelings of surprise, relief, thankfulness and joy that came over me. He was grinning from ear to ear; he even helped put my bags in the trunk. I gave him the biggest hug. I couldn't let him leave without mentioning the bill I told him, "Tommy, I don't know how you got this done without me paying for the parts, but I promise you I'll make payments every week for doing this for me." His reply was unbelievable

He said, "There is no bill. Now go and enjoy your family." I didn't know what to say. I'm thinking there is no bill? But how? I stood there in shock and Tommy got into the car that was waiting for him, smiled and waived to me. I waived back.

I got into my car, buckled my belt, reached over and buckled the belt in the passenger's seat and said out loud, "Buckle up, Jesus, we're going to Florida." It was the smoothest ride from beginning to end, the weather was absolutely gorgeous and my jaws ached from smiling. I remember hitting Tampa around 3pm which meant I could make it to my mom's work in Venice by the time she left for the day at 5pm. Sure enough I pulled up at 4:45pm; I walk into the shop and stood behind her customer with a big smile. You wouldn't believe the scream she let out when she saw my reflection in the mirror. It was awesome. My dad was due any moment to pick her up, so we arranged for me to be in her chair as if I were a customer when he walked in. I held a magazine up until I heard his foot steps near me. I dropped the magazine and coolly said, "Well, hello?" He quickly looked over and just as coolly replied, "Well, hello?" (You can never catch that man off guard). Despite his cool demeanor, when we walked outside he was so excited and started asking me questions "Why didn't you call?"

"How did you get here?" I wanted to tell him all I had been through in the days leading up to my surprise visit, but since we were about to leave I summarized it "All I can say is, I'm here Dad and it is a gift from God! That transmission in my car came from God! That is the only explanation; this trip is truly, truly a gift."

We hurried home so that I could see my brothers David was home and as soon as I walked in, he was hugging and kissing me hello. I asked where Sean was, my surprise couldn't be complete until I had seen Sean. Sean is super affectionate he would give me these bear hugs & he would squeeze my breath away.

David said he should be pulling up in a second. The words no sooner left his lips when the door opened and Sean came in. As soon as I saw him I started to cry. He hugged me and hugged me I cried and cried. I was happy, but it was the oddest feeling that I had. I couldn't understand why I was crying, almost weeping. I know everyone was accepting this as happy tears, but, in my mind, it didn't feel like happy tears. I specifically remember feeling a difference in my emotions greeting Sean verses the greeting I just had with my parents and David. It was notably odd.

Testimony-An Angel with a Map!

The following year and somewhere between 1992 & 1993, I made another solo trip to Florida. This one wasn't a surprise visit. The arrangements were seamless; however, the return to North Carolina wasn't so. I think I mentioned earlier that I'm not a seasoned traveler. So, this time I had a passenger with me, a little kitten that wandered into my apartment complex that I had adopted. "Precious" was her name and she accompanied me. It was a nice visit I had just enough money on me for the trip, gas, but nothing extra. I didn't want my family to worry, so when my parents asked me if I needed a few bucks, I quickly rejected it as my way of assuring them I was OK. On the return to North Carolina, as I was nearing the section in Georgia where I was supposed to exit I-75, for whatever reason, I decided to not exit I-75. I was making pretty good time, but it was getting dark and the weather started looking bad. I continued on I-75, as it began to pour down rain. Shame on me for not checking the wipers, now when I needed them the most, they didn't work! I was watching for signs for a decent gas station to turn into when I saw a sign that made my heart sink. It said "100 miles to Chattanooga." I thought, "Oh my God,

Chattanooga? That's in Tennessee!" I started to freak out, I was nearly on empty, had no money, it was pouring rain with wipers that didn't work, it was getting dark, I was hungry and now I find out I'm more than three hours from home. I was in a mess. "Oh Lord, please help me out of this one. Thank you for the visit to Florida, but I'm tired, hungry, broke and scared." I pull up to a pay phone (yes, a pay phone, cell phones were not big yet) and called my dad. They were expecting my call at that time (and I should have been telling them I was home); but I had to tell him the truth. I was so relieved to hear his voice and told my father what a stupid mistake I made by not exiting I-75 and now I was outside Tennessee! He tried to help me but he didn't have a map. I told him not to worry though I knew he would anyway, that I was at a gas station and I would get directions. I told them I would call as soon as I got home.

I sat there a few minutes to collect my thoughts. I went though my purse and the glove box for loose change and scrounged up 55 cents and put it into the tank. (No, I didn't have a credit card). I didn't want to use up any extra fuel so I didn't use the heater, in case that made a difference. I wasn't sure which direction I should begin so I thought to myself, "The next person

I see, I'll ask for directions." Up drives an older man in a little white pick-up truck. I walked over to him, he was wearing white overalls and I said, "Excuse me, Sir, but would you know how to get to Andrews from here?" He said "Andrews? That's in North Carolina" I said "Yes, I know I live there but I didn't take the exit off I-75 and wound up here, my wipers don't work, I'm just trying to get home." He could tell I wasn't a traveler and told me to hang on a minute. He went to his truck and returned with a map. He began giving me point specific directions (the kind of directions a girl like me needs to have); beginning with, "You'll take a left out of here" My mind was thinking about how I got myself into this mess I was barely listening to the man when suddenly he spoke to me in a very familiar way, the way my father had talked to me when I was growing up, the man's voice sounded just like my dad, He said, "Are you paying attention to me?" It was the oddest thing. He repeated "You'll take a left out of here, go up 1/2 mile and make a right and stay on that road until you see signs to the Ocoee." As soon as he said "Ocoee" I knew I was headed into the right direction I knew where the Ocoee & Nantahala Rivers were! He let me take his map and I was on my way. I didn't know if I would have enough gas, but I couldn't worry about it.

I kept thanking God for my meeting that man and how nice he was to give me his map. I began to wonder, "What would a man in Tennessee be doing with a map of North Carolina?" I made it back home in just less than three hours. I called my parents, who were near panicked. I assured them I was fine and told them that I met an angel and he guided me in.

* * *

Writing a book is hard, believe it or not. You get an idea and get in the groove of writing it out. Once you are finished with that idea you realize that section will make more sense in another area (along the same subject) so....you copy & paste. Then someone knocks on the door or the phone rings, so you leave the computer.....then you come back and find your 10 year old at the computer typing along. You sit down and realize the entire section you just spent 2 hours on has magically disappeared (one time the entire book disappeared!) Talk about being ticked! I've written this book nearly 3 times, for all of the reasons stated above. SO, if this book ever becomes a real book, it will be a miracle..... I just needed to get that out.☺

CHAPTER 2

Remember back when I was speaking with Pastor Hamilton in North Carolina? I mentioned that other things we discussed would come up later in the book. Well, on the day I spoke with Pastor Hamilton I had also discussed frustrations of being alone just as intently as I talked about my broken car. After I made the surprise visit to see my family in Florida, I returned to my everyday life in North Carolina. Three days after I got back I met the most wonderful guy. His name is Tim. He and I instantly became an item.

A group of tree trimmers came into our small town to do contract work.

Anyone who lived there would know "outsiders" when we see them, especially a pack of them running around everywhere together. One day I was washing my car at the do-it-yourself car wash and I was approached by four of the outsiders who were washing their vehicle. Two of them were named Tim, the bold one and the quiet one. The bold one had a ring on his finger and seemed to do the most flirting; the other guys were pleasantly courteous and friendly. We didn't talk about much and we didn't talk long. We exchanged "hi, how are you doing?", "nice weather we are having", "what is there to do around here?" stuff like that. And I went on my way. A few nights later a girlfriend was driving me around town when she made a stop at the town pool hall. We walked in and all of the out of town tree trimmers were there shooting pool. She and I quietly joked with each other about how nice looking one of them was. We didn't intend to stay, so we left. I noticed the good-looking one glancing in our direction, but maybe it was because I looked back at him?

A few nights later, I went up to the pizza place for my "to go" order and once again, this group of tree trimmers was hanging out there. The same bold chatterbox struck up a conversation with me, but this time I didn't take my eye off the good-looking one in the back seat of the car. This time there was no mistake he had his eye on me. We seemed to be having our own private conversation right there in front of everybody. As soon as my order was ready.....while looking directly at him and with a smile I said two words,"Get in." He said, "move over boys..." and proceeded to move the front seat out of his way, got out and sat in my car. I waved "bye" to the rest of his group and we drove off. Tim and I have been together ever since that night.

I guess I can say "I picked him up"!

Tim and I met in March 1993. I lived in North Carolina from 1989 until we moved back to Florida together late 1994.

We were engaged in Feb. 1996. He proposed to me the day before Valentine's! We were all so happy. In 1996 our poor families were put through the ringer with weddings! My brother Sean was married in April or May. Tim's sister Kelly and her boyfriend Chris were married in June and then Tim and I were married in September 1996.

I have hopes, I have faith and the Lord has given me these wonderful gifts. A loving, kind, generous, likable, hard working, loyal man. Not to mention all the necessary things needed in between, our loving families, our jobs, our home and life's essentials. I am blessed. We have had troubles, but we're still blessed.

After Tim and I had been dating a while, he brought me to meet his family in Cols, Georgia. His sister Kelly had taken me to the side and said something to me I will always treasure she told me she and her mom thought I was terrific for Tim and they were so glad that I was part of his life (something extremely sweet like that, I don't remember her exact words). I took what she meant very much to heart, as a sister who loves her brother. I was touched.

After several months and when it was certain Tim and I were in a relationship, we made a trip to Florida to meet my family. On the return drive home, we had a situation that we can only attribute to God and his love and care for us.

Testimony – A Family of Angels

We were driving my old black Buick, we were in the last couple hours of the 12 hour ride back to North Carolina, but we left Florida a lot later then I would have normally left had I been traveling solo. So by the 9th hour it was dark out. Not giving that any importance whatsoever until the car began to overheat. It was late December and the weather in North Carolina was pretty cold now and with it being late, dark and a very long & lonely road in North Carolina, we were a little worried.

Although we had already set plans for moving to Florida permanently we still had to pack our belongings and finalize moving arrangements. We didn't count on being stranded in the car for the night, but that's how it was beginning to look.

There was a container with a little water in it in the trunk, but it wasn't going to be enough to get us back to Andrews from were we were. Not many cars were on the road at all. We mostly noticed a few cars going in the opposite direction.

I began to worry that my parents would worry if I didn't call them soon. (These were the days before everyone had a cell phone.) I remember saying a prayer asking God to help us out of this I figured the worst would be us huddling for the night in the car, but I would never be able to sleep if I wasn't able to phone my folks. While Tim was rooting around in the trunk for anything he could find a car pulled up behind us. I was so thankful for having my handgun, but how do I protect my boyfriend who is outside in the open? Due to the headlights, I couldn't see who Tim was speaking to, but I heard another man's voice and then I thought I heard a baby crying. I got out of the car to sort out what I was hearing and I look over to Tim who gave me a reassuring look. I saw a few different figures inside the other vehicle, a woman holding a baby and three or four other kids in back. This immediately made me feel safe. As soon as I absorbed what I saw, Tim was gathering our belongings and asked me to lock up the car and come with him. The people were going to drive us to the nearest gas station. I was so glad

Tim was with me, I could never have done this if I were alone.

Within five minutes, we were at the gas station, but it was obviously closed. Not one person in site. The driver looked at his wife and asked us where we were headed. We told them we lived in Andrews, but we certainly didn't expect them to go so far out of their way so we were deciding if we should stay at the gas station or go back to the car, but the driver had already decided for us, they were there to help and he said it wasn't too far out of their way to take us to Andrews! I was positively shocked! Why would this man, take his entire family at 10:30-11PM on a two hour trip to Andrews and back? I can't describe the feelings of relief and appreciation that I felt, although I was still on "stranger guard." The man explained that it was "not a big deal". They were on there way to pay their mortgage which was on the way. I remember looking at Tim with "what in the world is going on?" eyes. He just shrugged his shoulders and patted me on the knee. A few seconds later the driver took this quick little turn, onto this bumpy dirt road. I immediately went into "oh crap" mode. I was in a total panic thinking we were about to be taken hostage and cut up into pieces. I dug my fingernails into Tim's leg. He gave me a smile and patted my knee.

I can't remember if Tim asked or if the man volunteered this information, but the driver apologized for the bumpy road and said they had to make a little stop to pay their mortgage. (Oh yeah, I think I remember someone saying something about paying the mortgage.) I would never have figured a building would be back where he was driving, but sure enough about 10 minutes into this bumpy-dirt road was a wide, cleared area and what appeared to be a small bank! The man jumped out, put an envelope into the slot and we were on our way back to the main highway. About 45 minutes later he pulled up to my apartment. We tried giving the driver the few dollars we had on us, to repay them in gas, but the man wouldn't hear of it. I asked the man for his name and city where they live, so that I could send them a note of thanks and I also wanted to tell my pastor of their kindness, how grateful we were for their assistance with all the circumstances. To this day, Tim and I refer to them as that "the family of angels."

CHAPTER 3

I've been quoted saying "1998 was a year from hell." I shouldn't say it that way really because it's also the year we had our first beautiful girl. But, she, in fact, was the only light that year.

I surprised my husband and parents around Christmas time 1997 with the news that I was expecting. I remember the day I found out I was pregnant like it was yesterday. It was a Saturday afternoon, Tim and I were going to his company Christmas party that evening. I was home cleaning house and waiting for him to come home from work. I bought a home pregnancy test the day before, not really believing I could be pregnant. I was home alone and took the test. After seeing the positive result and flipping out I sat there in my bedroom on the edge of the bed scared, numb, overwhelmed but just so happy. I was determined to tell Tim first. I held back all impulses to call Michele, my dearest girlfriend, and especially not my mom. I had to tell Mom in person. I wanted to see her reaction I wanted to tell her so badly, but this was special and Tim had to know first. I decided to make both Tim and my mom Christmas cards I felt like the news was a present to me and I wanted it to be a present to them too. I paced the floor waiting for Tim to get home, it was agonizing.

I printed up the cards on the computer, got ready for the party and it felt like an eternity waiting for my husband to get home from work. He walked in and kissed me hello, he sees I'm all dressed for the party.....I start to hand him the card and he politely asks me if it can wait. He wanted to wash the car before the sun went down. So I wait.

He comes back inside. I stand up grinning from ear to ear, hand him the card and, again, he politely asks me if it can wait. He wanted to jump in the shower. So I wait. He's finally done, I hand him the card, it said something mushy about how much we've been through, how much I love him, "its Christmas time, and you're going to be a daddy." It was so funny, simultaneously his eyes practically bugged-out of his head, he yells 'WHAT!" and he jerked his neck from reading the card to looking up at me in 0.5 seconds. After hugs there were tears and I told him he had to hurry up and drive me over to my parent's house or I would explode after holding in this news all day. Having to wait for him to wash the car and then shower killed me.

We get to my parents' house and, to my surprise, both my brothers were there. I was so happy to be able to tell everyone in person. My mom read her card; she lets out a scream and jumps up to hug me. Both my brothers come quickly into the kitchen, nearly ready to draw their weapons – after hearing my mom shout. Everyone's reactions were just so cool.

In May of '98, while my parents were visiting relatives in New York, my dad had a heart attack. At the time he didn't seek medical attention. They flew back home to Florida (a big no-no due to air pressure changes) and almost immediately after landing my mom had him in the hospital being checked out. He learned that he had 90-something percent blockage in his arteries and he would need open heart surgery. All of us were in a panic of worry. The surgeon said he would need a triple bypass. He would have his surgery in the next two weeks.

My brothers, polar opposites but each with a very special and loving bond with our dad, both wore the news on their face. All of us were thinking, "Is this Dad's time?" I think Sean, the youngest and especially close to Dad took the news the hardest. Dad is Sean's hero. Dad is like John Wayne in Sean's eyes. He mimics Dad in almost every way, from the movies they enjoy, the food they eat, the guns they collect, the books, the cars and even music. They also resemble each other physically.

Dad sits with Sean for hours and he tells all the stories of his upbringing in Brooklyn, the times dad hung out with his friends (a real bunch of wise guys; they called themselves "the Parkside Saints"), and dad tells him details about the elaborate parties during his drinking years, the card games, stories about the neighborhood. He would throw around some impressive names. It is practically a story straight out of "The Bronx Tale" mixed with a little of "The Godfather" and "Casino." Sean can never get enough of it and I know how proud Sean is of Dad. Dad always gets a kick out of reminiscing by way of Sean and the charge it gives him seeing Sean's enthusiasm and compelling interest. They are each other's confidants. Sometimes their conversations make their way into the living room and Mom will add what she remembered, like the time Dad called her in the middle of the night to tell her he was sitting next to Rosemary Clooney having a drink and John Carradine was also there. We kids were totally wowed by the story, but for mom being awakened at 2:30am for any reason didn't go over well. All of us would talk and laugh for hours, longer if we had any guests. Our love of one another and being with each other is generally known and absolutely unconditional. The phrase "we're a close family" doesn't quite describe us I think we're closer than close.

In June '98 Dad underwent his bypass surgery. I took the day off to be with my mother in the waiting room. David and Sean waited at home. It was an intense day and I was in charge of keeping the rest of the family (aunts, uncles & grandparents) informed. When the surgeon came out to speak to us, he was confident and direct; Dad did extremely well and was in recovery but he added that his triple bypass wound up being a six-way bypass once they opened him up! We asked if we could see him and the surgeon said we could. Dad would be heavily sedated and wouldn't even know we were there, but both Mom and I had to see him. The nurse came out to escort us to ICU, to me; she appeared to have a look of concern on her face. I asked her if my dad was really OK and she assured me that he was, but I found out her concern was for mom and me, seeing him. She warned us that he was hooked up to machines and there were tubes, etc. I was relieved but insisted that we didn't care what he looked like, we needed to see him. We soon realized that when a nurse says she is concerned about what one witnesses, one should listen to the nurse. She tried to prepare us, but nothing could prepare us. We took two steps into the room and I immediately thought I would faint. My father looked positively dead. He was white as a ghost with giant tubes in his mouth, machines making Darth Vader breathing noises, lying there lifeless. We both immediately begin crying, moving toward him. I touched his hand as Mom leaned in and gave him a kiss. Anyway we find out he should be in a room in several hours. We quickly decide to take a break, let dad wake up and I will phone family to give them an update.... and we would come back. I'll never forget... when I called my brother David to give him the good news that Dad was out of surgery and was doing fine. At the moment I started to cry. He asked me why I was so upset. I tried to tell him I think it was the mixture of emotions running through my head, fright, relief and heartbreak upon seeing Dad in that hospital room, I couldn't really explain it. David says "Your eyes saw something you weren't supposed to see". All I could say was, "yes, we both did".

As dad recuperated from surgery, I was half way into my 7th month of pregnancy and I was getting bigger and bigger. I was so thankful and very fortunate to not have any complications with the pregnancy. We tried being happy, but my dad's heart attack and his surgery was a pretty big distraction.

My mom planned a *wonderful* surprise baby shower for me in June of that year. It was lovely my closest friends and family were there. I was about to find out, however, that a roller coaster of emotions had only just begun.

The following Saturday afternoon Tim was outside playing around in the garage and was messing with the car window. We had been having trouble with the driver side window; it had slipped. He was busy taking the door panel off to fix it and I was inside on the couch taking a nap. All of a sudden, he rushes into the house (with one of those voices you don't hear very often) and says "Baby, we have to go to the hospital". I was in total relaxation mode and said, "No, honey. I'm fine, really. The baby isn't coming right now, I'm fine". He said (with that voice)...."No, we have to go now". He is holding what appeared to be a red towel, his hand held straight up. I soon realize it was, in fact, a white rag that was soaked and dripping in blood. You've never seen a 7 ½ month pregnant woman move so fast, I jumped up, grabbed the keys and said "Get in the truck! I'll drive!"

So, I'm driving and asking him all kinds of questions. "Oh my God, are you ok?" "What the hell did you do?" He was afraid to tell me, thinking the news would make me go into labor or something. After going back and forth a little, he decided to tell me he cut his finger off. Apparently, there is thin sheet metal in the door panel, he had pliers in his hand and was trying to pull something out of the door panel and with the force of his pulling, the pliers slipped, when the pliers slipped his hand kept moving and did so, just right into the side of the sheet metal. Now I'm getting a little panicked, wondering if it his finger was there, or left at the house and disturbing things like this. Somehow he was able to tell me it was there, but barely. He refused to let me see it.

We got to the hospital and they took him right in. They needed to call in a plastic surgeon, someone able to reconnect arteries. He basically needed to have his finger reattached.

Talk about an eventful day, but, thank God Tim's finger was saved. It was pretty sore and he would need to have rehabilitation, but he still had 10 fingers.

CHAPTER 4

Ok so, its summer 1998 and my dad was still recuperating from major open heart surgery, my husband recuperating from cutting his finger off two days ago and I'm nearly 8 months pregnant with our first baby! I'm driving home from work and decided to stop at my parent's house to check on my dad. He's sitting on the couch, on the phone. I walk in, I wave "hi" he waves back and gives me a raised eyebrow. I go about my business but I can tell he's in an intense conversation. Well, he was listening intently. He hangs up the phone and explains that he was speaking with my mom who is at the hospital with my brother Sean, Sean's wife and my brother David.

Sean had recently been having bizarre symptoms of headaches and his equilibrium was off and on this day Sean's doctor had him go to the hospital for a CT scan. The doctor walked into the room, so that's why my mom hung up with my dad. So my Dad fills me in about the situation.

I'm wondering why I hadn't heard about Sean feeling bad until now when the phone rings. Dad picks it right up and I can tell it's my mom's chatter. As I'm watching my dad his expression suddenly disappears and I immediately get a feeling of panic over me. What could she possibly say to make him look this way? Then I hear him say, "In his brain?" I remember feeling numb and I felt like shouting "What's with whose brain? Stop talking and tell me what's going on!", however, he needed to listen to what he was being told. When he hung up he tells me that Sean had the CT scan and they saw what appears to be a brain tumor. I asked him if they knew if it was cancerous. He said they are going to run more tests but they will probably refer him to Shands Hospital in Gainesville for further testing.

I sat there frozen. Maybe it was shock. All I know is I had thousands of questions but couldn't speak. I couldn't imagine how hard this was for my parents. They were obviously worried about Sean, but my dad's health was extremely fragile. They were worried about the added stress on me and the baby as I was just into my 8th month. We were deeply concerned for Sean and for what this could be. He was a new father with a 14-month-old son.

Unfortunately, several days later my brother

Sean was diagnosed with probably the rarest type of brain cancer (Atypical Rhabdoid). It had been found in only a couple previous cases all of which were children and each under the age of two, with no survivors. There were many long discussions; one doctor mentioned Sean could have had this in his head lying dormant all these years.

While this is going on, a friend of mine Darlene, (a single mom of three; ages 7 ½, 10 & 11) found out that her middle son, Josh (10) had a brain tumor. Josh was in All Children's Hospital in Tampa and was having surgery to remove the tumor and they would then run tests to see if it was malignant. I was very pregnant at the time and had a lot going on with my family. Against my families wishes I drove to Tampa to show my support and prayed for mercy for Josh. We were relieved to learn Josh's tumor was benign.

Three months after Sean's diagnosis and on the day he was having his 3rd cranial operation, I went into labor. My mom and I had planned on her being my coach in the delivery room (with my husband); but with Sean being so fragile, I insisted that my parents stay with him until they were certain he was stable. In the meantime my Aunt Marian (Marian Owen, my mom's sister) came to be with me and Tim at the hospital. It was supposed to be a happy time for me and Tim, but I was absolutely crushed inside thinking about my brother fighting for his life.

My parents were in Gainesville waiting for Sean to come out of surgery. Once he was out of recovery my parents began the drive from Gainesville to Sarasota. Mom wanted to try to make it for the delivery. I can't imagine the emotions and stress they were under. The emotional rollercoaster. I was also worried that all the tension, lack of sleep and anxiety could cause my dad to have a setback. He had just had open heart surgery! I wasn't sure who I was supposed to focus on. This was enough "fuel" of stress to travel to the moon.

While I was in labor, the baby was apparently giving the nurses cause for concern. They were trying to keep it from me as much as they could, but when little bells start going off and 30 people come rushing into the room, it kind of let the cat out of the bag. Our baby's heart rate kept dropping with every contraction, and it would plummet when I would push – I didn't know it at the time, but the cord was wrapped around the baby's neck.

The doctor came in to check on me and said if the baby didn't come soon they would have to give me a C-section. Under no circumstances did I want surgery; my family had been through enough surgeries. I remember telling the doctor, "Tell me what to do and I'll do it". They were gearing me up and just as we were about to begin I heard a nurse say; "Kim's mother is here." I couldn't believe it. I thought they were in Gainesville with Sean. There was a controversy about having too many people in the room (spouse, Aunt and now mom) and without hesitating, Aunt Marian walked out so that my mom could stay in. I was so happy to see her and immediately asked how Sean was. She told me he made it through surgery just fine and was awake and speaking to them when they left.

Almost as if her presence was the ingredient missing, with my husband and now my mom by my side, we delivered our precious Heather Rae, 6.6oz. Mom made it just in time. We opted to not know the baby's gender until delivery. I can still hear my mom's voice yelling, "Kim, it's a GIRL, IT'S A GIRL!!"

After four long months of tears, hopes, prayers, traveling back & forth to Gainesville, four fragile cranial operations, positive reports, negative reports, numerous tests & biopsies, more prayers, operations, sickness, seizures, intense stereotactic radiation therapy our beloved Sean lost his battle with brain cancer on Nov. 24, 1998. That day my dad lost his buddy, my mom lost a bright star in her life, David lost his friend....his little brother and I lost a precious friend...my little brother. It was just so very hard on all of us. Just as hard on us now, but I think we deal with it better. I (we) are so very thankful to God for His guidance throughout the crisis; even though my family had to endure ruthless, hurtful and extremely unnecessary frustrations on top of dealing with my brother's illness. God brought us peace. God helped us through, I believe that with my heart and I feel time does heal.

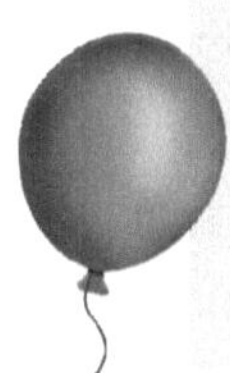

Remembering a kind and gentle soul,
a very special man:
Sean McAuliffe lost his battle with
cancer Nov. 24, 1998

I came across this story prior to my brother's passing:

We often learn the most from our children. Some time ago, a friend of mine punished his 3-year old daughter for wasting a roll of gold wrapping paper. Money was tight, and he became infuriated when the child tried to decorate a box to put under the tree. Nevertheless, the little girl brought the gift to the father the next morning and said, "This is for you Daddy".

He was embarrassed by his earlier overreaction, but his anger flared again when he found that the box was empty. He yelled at her, "Don't you know that when you give someone a present, there's supposed to be something inside of it?"

The little girl looked up at him with tears in her eyes and said, "Oh Daddy, it's not empty. I blew kisses into the box. All for you Daddy." The father was crushed. He put his arms around his little girl, and he begged her forgiveness.

He kept that gold box by his bed for years. Whenever he was discouraged, he would take out an imaginary kiss & remember the love of the child who had put it there.

In a very real sense, each of us as parents has been given a gold container filled with unconditional love and kisses from our children. There is no more precious possession anyone could hold.

After reading this, the thought entered my mind, if I were going to lose my brother, how wonderful it would be to always have a kiss from him, and to share them with the people I love & the people he loves.

At first I didn't know how I was going to get him to kiss a box without him raising questions that would be difficult to answer.

I went to the drug store to buy a few greeting cards and bought small some boxes. I was on my way to Sean's house and decided to bring the bag of boxes inside with me. Sean and dad were watching a movie (American Graffiti to be exact), I casually said "Hey pal, do me a favor and blow some kisses into this bag". I held open the bag & without asking me one question, he blew kisses in the bag. I thanked him, closed the bag & he continued to watch the movie. Sean died two days later.

The night he passed away, I proceeded to put the boxes together.

I opened all the boxes, shook the bag up a bit to multiply the kisses and I poured out the kisses into the boxes – filling each box up. Then I typed up labels.

The outside of all the boxes read "Butterfly Kisses" and the top of the box says "Open when you need a kiss from Sean". Inside the box top also has a personalized message, each slightly different, like, mine says:

"I love you Kim
I know you love me
Don't be sad
We will be together again
I will wait for you,

Your brother,
Sean"

During the funeral I gave out the boxes. One to my dad, my mom, David, a couple of Sean's closest friends, wife, his son, my grandparents and I think some Aunts and Uncles too.

It feels so good knowing each box has genuine kisses of his inside. I call them "forever kisses".

If you think that is neat. I was able to do this more than once. I'll explain later on.

CHAPTER 5

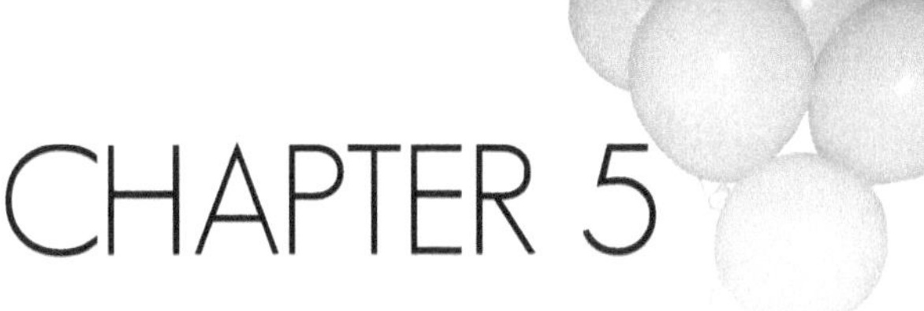

A test of faith. It must have been the 2nd week of March 2003. Tim and I were overjoyed to learn we were expecting again. I remember we were "not trying" but that we were "not preventing" either.

We made a mistake of telling our 4 year old she was going to have a little brother or sister soon. See below in my log of "things Heather does".

- Age 3 – Heather can recite the Lord's Prayer by herself.

- Age 4 – Heather can tie her shoes.

- April 26, 2003. Heather is 4 years old and I'm 6 weeks along with #2.

- This is my log of "things Heather says & does".... That I promised my mom I would write down.

- 2 weeks ago when we woke Heather to get ready to go to Miss Pat's (the babysitter) she said "mommy, mommy I need a drink of water...and hurry!" I said, "OK, I'll get you some water but why the big hurry?" She said, "Because I think I swallowed a bug and it bit my throat!"

- After learning we were expecting #2, we told Heather the news. She seemed pleased to learn that she'll have a little brother or sister soon. Each day we talk with her a little bit about it, reinforcing all the positives, "You'll be the big sister..."; "you'll be a big help to mommy & daddy...", "how much we're going to love the baby..." and "how much the baby will love us..." Then, with Heather on my lap, I was telling her that the baby is right here in my belly right now, and can hear us and loves us already! Heather said "Mommy quick open your mouth real wide, like this (she opened her mouth). Thinking the conversation was over and we were playing a game, I proceeded to open my mouth. Heather leaned over and yells in my mouth "HELLO BABY, I LOVE YOU!"

- One day we stopped at the local circle K store to pick up a lottery ticket, my husband who was driving and Heather in the back seat wait for me in the car. While in the store and with

Easter only a few days away I notice a display of Easter Bunny Pez dispensers. I picked one out for Heather, got my ticket and was on my way. When I sat down in the car, I tossed Heather her new toy. She replies, "Oh mommy, now I know you must really love me!"

I had hoped to have a sibling for Heather when she was 4. It just seemed like a decent age difference. It was important to me for her to be close to her sibling, the way both Tim and I are with our siblings.

I wish I was able to recall all the fluffy feelings and actions that took place. I have no doubt I jumped around like a happy fool, called my friends and family – the whole routine......but sadly on May 8, 2003 I miscarried.

I had taken a home pregnancy test and called my doctor. They gave me an appointment and so by the appointment day I would be in my 9th week. They were going to check everything & listen to the heart beat. Tim came with me to the appointment and he waited in the lobby.

While the nurse is looking around for the heart beat, this heat wave of panic came over me as I looked up at her face. I'm laying there waiting for her to say something, but she just kept searching and searching. Finally she said "oh

 Kim Clark

honey.....there isn't a heart beat". They estimated
I must have lost the baby during my 5th week
and I just didn't know it.

They called Tim into the room; we were both
crushed and just so sad. I asked for answers but
all the doctor would say was its unexplained, it
happens all the time but they can't give direct answer as to why it happens. The reassurances we
were given by people were things like, there was
probably something wrong with the baby and so
it couldn't develop into full term, but it's probably a good thing or you could have had a child
with a disability. Useless comforts like this.

We did our best to pick ourselves up. I remember going to church looking for comfort, understanding anything to shake this crushing feeling. This one morning, we all got dressed, drove
to church, said hello to my parents and sat down.
The minute I heard the music, I began to cry, we
got up and we left. I couldn't go to church. We
didn't go for several weeks. I wasn't angry with
God, but I was angry. It hurt, all the time.

I wanted what I lost and we thought if I got
pregnant again this intense sadness would go
away.

We not only dealt with intense sadness and
very hopeless and helpless feelings, we endured
2 additional years of infertility.

We both went through tests and blood work. There wasn't anything wrong with either one of us. It was simply not in God's plan for us to have another child and part of me couldn't accept that.

Each month we put ourselves on a schedule. It was miserable.

After a while the overwhelming "I must get pregnant" feeling began to subside. I became more accepting (which I believe is the Holy Spirit). That led into feelings of satisfaction. We were both absolutely and totally, one hundred percent satisfied and thankful having one beautiful, active, healthy child.

I put away the ovulation calendar and decided to end this monthly mechanical routine indefinitely. We were free from this monster and instead we loved each other.

Then, June 8, 2005 I found out I was pregnant. And February 8th we welcomed little Michele. Michele Bea (she is named after my dearest friend Michele DelMonaco and Bea is after my grandmother Beatrice. And I have an Aunt Bea (Brooklyn Bea Hansen). We sometimes call Michele Shelby.

What frustrates me was it took 2 years to find out not every woman ovulates between day 14 & 18 (whatever it is)....some of us (obviously) ovulate early, like day 8!!

What this taught me was. Sometimes what we truly want we may be capable of as long as God wants that for you as well.

Matthew 6:33-34 But seek ye first his kingdom and his righteousness, and all these things will be given to you as well. Therefore do not worry about tomorrow, for tomorrow will worry about itself. Each day has enough trouble of its own.

Remember back when I was in labor with Heather? I told you how my Aunt Marian came to be with Tim & me in the hospital? And then when my mom showed up there was an issue with 3 people being in the room with me, so my Aunt had stepped out? Well, I never forgot how gracious she was to do that after spending nearly 18 hours with us and at the last minute she wasn't able to witness the birth.

I had always told Tim, if I ever got pregnant again, I would invite Aunt Marian to the delivery. Well, that's exactly what we did! I even sent her an invitation. It wound up being a wonderful memory for all of us and my mom got to witness the birth of her second granddaughter with her sister.

CHAPTER 6

In early Jan. 2008 I felt like I was beginning to get a sore throat. It became something I noticed each morning and then I began to notice it during the day.

On top of that I began feeling extremely tired, constantly. Even on the weekends and even after taking a nap. I couldn't understand it. I ate well, took vitamins and I would rest.

February 2, 2008 I woke with the most painful feeling in my chest. It was my first time ever having heart burn, but that's the only words I can use to describe it. My chest was on fire and at times I could not move. I needed to put the fire out so I got a tall glass of ice water and began to sip it, slow but steady. After about 20 seconds I thought I would explode. It felt like the water I just drank had turned to lava and was about to boil out. It was so painful I told Tim if I kept feeling like this I should go to the hospital.

Within the next 30 minutes we were on our way to the hospital in Port Charlotte. We get to the hospital and they immediately gave me a chest X-ray, an EKG and blood work. After several hours the ER doctor comes in to tell me I had acid reflux, we should be sure to slightly elevate the head of our bed and he prescribed antacids. We went home.

I was relieved. I continued to perform my every day routines but bizarre things began to happen. The strange feeling in my throat was still happening too. But it wasn't sore; it actually never got sore, it felt more like a lump after I would swallow.

I went to see our primary physician who works with a physicians group in Osprey. I'll call him *Dr. Queen.* I first began seeing Dr. Queen many years ago, at least 10 years before we had Heather and she was now 10. He was the girls' and my primary physician.

So, he checks me out and didn't find anything wrong with me or with my throat, but I told him I felt something in my throat. As long as I wasn't in pain, he didn't seem overly concerned.

It suddenly seemed like I had to see the doctor every time I would turn around! Not only for myself but for the kids too. I can look back at records and show you tons of doctor's visits. Some of these reasons seemed unbelievable and outrageous! I felt like a complete hypochondriac.

Feb. 7, 2008 – I saw a Chiropractor for excruciating pain in my shoulders & neck.

Mar. 6, 2008 – (my birthday) I saw Dr. Queen – Michele had a virus – I mentioned the lump in my throat.

Mar. 10, 2008 – Went to Dr.Queen – Michele still had the virus & now I had it.

Mar. 13, 2008 – I saw Dr.Queen for unbelievable fatigue. He said something like "well you are over 40 with 2 kids and kids do take a lot out of you especially working full time".

Mar. 27, 2008 – I woke up with painful and very swollen ankles! Who does this happen to? I saw Dr. Queen for the swollen ankles & fatigue "very impressive" he said. He examined my throat, I requested an x-ray, and he said we'll keep an eye on it. He prescribed anti inflammatory meds & sent me home.

Apr. 1, 2008 – Heather had strep throat; we saw Dr. Queen's nurse practioner and I told her about the lump in my throat.

Apr. 11, 2008 – I saw Dr. Queen (I forget why, but I paid a co-pay).

Apr. 15, 2008 – I saw the nurse practitioner for fatigue and the lump in my throat was much worse. She said she and Dr. Queen consulted, they will start tests & I may see a rheumatologist, I asked about having an x-ray of my neck.

Apr. 16, 2008 – I had blood work to check my thyroid. I requested blood work for my heart; I will have to fast tonight and have blood taken in the am.

Apr. 17, 2008 – I woke with a severely swollen neck, difficulty breathing, husband rushed me back to the hospital in Port Charlotte. I explained I was there in Feb.; I had a chest X-ray, EKG & blood work (and now this). I explain my primary discussed sending me to a rheumatologist. ER doc didn't feel he should put me through tests, only to be repeated so he prescribed pain meds for my neck & we went home.

Apr. 18, 2008 – I saw Dr. Queen for neck and join pains. I asked for more attention on my throat/neck as the lump was feeling very pronounce and it is interfering with eating and my breathing, it's getting worse.

The situation in my throat started to worry me as I began to feel like I was being choked. I could turn my neck a certain way and when I did I wasn't able to breathe. I remember one night that I sat straight up in the bed; I was awakened by gasping for air.

Apr. 28, 2008 – I saw the nurse practitioner for post nasal drip and this never ending lump in my throat. She examined my throat/neck; said she thinks I should see a GI specialist, and it might take a few weeks to get in. A few weeks? I flipped out and demanded an immediate picture, scan, something of my neck! I said "I don't care if it's an X-ray, MRI or a "blank-ing" Polaroid; I want a picture of my neck! I want it now, I can't breathe!!!"

My appointment was in 2 days. When I was leaving the doctor's office a nice lady named Renee noticed my "permanent make up" sign on my truck. We chatted a few minutes and set up an appointment for Saturday, May 3rd.

Apr. 29, 2008 – I woke with severe jaw pain &/or pain in my left ear – it was hard to tell. Saw my dentist. He examined the area, tapped on every tooth but was unable to determine where the pain was coming from. I was miserable.

May 1, 2008 – I arrive at the GI specialist's office for this CT scan, extremely nervous. I was up all night worried they will find something. I walk up to the counter and I hear this cheerful voice "Hi, isn't your name Kim?" I was so in thought I really wasn't expecting to see someone I knew. I said yes. She said 'I thought so; I'm Melissa we went to high school together!". Right there, God put her there. A familiar face, his hand. This is what I'm talking about! I needed comforts, He provided it.

May 6, 2008 – I had to undergo a biopsy (details will follow shortly) – I'm a wreck of nerves because they have to put me to sleep. My husband and parents are with me and we walk into this enormous facility and we're busy looking for the suite when I notice this extremely familiar face walking towards me. I swear I know this guy, but why can't I place him. As he gets closer it hits me – it's Dennis! The UPS guy that comes to my office every single day! It took me a second to recognize him because he was in street clothes. We said hello, we stop to chat and exchange reasons why each of us are there, we said good bye and we go back about our business. Right there, God provided me a comfort I deeply needed. He provided another familiar face.

CHAPTER 7

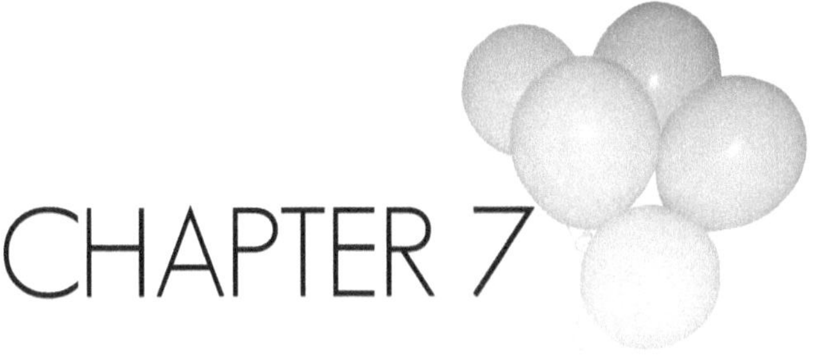

These e-mails will explain what was going on.

5-7-08

Hello e-mail friends;

Some of you may already know, but to those who don't; I have a bit of challenging news.

For the last few months I've been having bizarre medical symptoms and kept visiting the doctor.

I had a CT scan on May 1, 2008 and was told on Friday 2nd that I have Lymphoma. (Diffuse Large B Cell Lymphoma, non-Hodgkin)

It's treatable, it's curable, and it's survivable. I have a mass in my chest above my heart that is pressing against my esophagus. It's 10cm by 6cm – which is large.

Last Monday they scanned my abdomen, chest & pelvis and were able to confirm the mass is isolated to my chest/neck, which is good news.

I had a biopsy on Tuesday which confirmed the CT scans findings, it is Lymphoma.

I'm having a PET scan tomorrow and they will discuss all test results and treatment with us on Monday 12th.

We are confident in our faith and have received great encouragement & strength since we got the news.

From our loving families & friends; though their prayers and positive reinforcement. It means a lot and it works.

Please keep us in your prayers. We'll do our best to send out updates as this unfolds.

Love,
Kim and family.....who are, have been and will continue to be in God's hands.

May 3rd (Saturday) – this entry is not a doctor's appointment, believe it or not. I had made the make up appointment with Renee outside my primary doctor's office. She came to my studio in North Port for eye liner. I was late to the appointment but my father was there to let her in and to begin her paperwork. He found her to be delightful.

He tells her about my diagnosis and that we were just told the news yesterday. She tells him that she had lung cancer and even had one lung removed. She spoke to him in a manner of such hope and comfort; he felt she was there to give us a very important message.

I wasn't in any mood to be working, but I made the appointment and figured the distraction (away from having cancer) would do me good.

I finally arrive and can't get over how happy my dad looks. Renee looks up at me and said, "your dad was telling me all about your news from yesterday and honey you are going to be just fine". I felt like crying. I look over and my dad is smiling. Renee and I exchanged stories and the more I listened to her, the more comfort I felt. I told her I thought she was an angel. She had this way of making us see this grim situation not look so hopeless. We were dealing with Lymphoma, not lung cancer, not brain cancer. Not that Lymphoma is a walk through the park, but maybe a lot of our feelings were based on having lost Sean to cancer. We had only just gotten this news and none of us knew what it meant or what to expect. There was so much we still had to find out.

After I begin to work on Renee, my mom showed up. I was happy she was able to meet

Renee and mom also got the comforts she needed. Mom thought she was an angel. (Great minds think alike). One thing is certain, God lead Renee there.

The next time you dine at the Dutch Valley Restaurant in Sarasota, tell Renee (Owner) "Kim thinks you are an angel!"

5-13-08

Hello again,

Monday we met with the Oncologist and received an absolute ton of information and a surprise bone marrow test.

I have type B – large cell lymphoma (non-Hodgkin's); his guess is stage 2 but won't know definitely until results of the bone marrow come back. It would be nice to hear stage 2; but even if the marrow test supports stage 4 the treatment will be the same they say, so they are not as focused on staging in this type of cancer. So they said.

Their prognosis is very positive and treatment begins this Wednesday 14th at 11:30am (takes 2 hours). I go Thursday for another regimen (that takes 6-7 hours!) & may have a shot of something-or-other on Friday.

I have a boatload of prescriptions to take...those

who know me, know I try to limit how much meds I take, but now things are different and everything they prescribe is regimented. I will do what they recommend, but can't help myself when I see a police officer…. I feel like I should turn myself in!! ☺

I'll have chemo Wed., & another process on Thursday & possibly 1 shot on Friday. Then I'll be done for 3 weeks. They say I'll feel "flu like" symptoms a couple of days after the chemo. I will repeat these steps every third week for a cycle of 6. (Almost 5 months). I'll say bye-bye to my hair two weeks after chemo. Hair will be back two months after chemo ends.

Again we are grateful for the love & support system we have; I'm blessed to have God guiding me though, I've already been picked up by a few angels that have "shown up" just prior to & since this trial begun. I feel like there is a purpose for all of this and unfortunately there are others who are having harder struggles.

Sorry for the blanket e-mail, I'm sure you know it's a lot easier to update everyone at once via e-mail.

Thank you all for your prayers!

Much love always,
Kim & family

Fri. 5-16-08

Hi ya......Medicated mama here;
On Wednesday 14th – treatment 1st day

Tim & my parents didn't know this, but I wore a Howard Stern wig to work, before treatment at 11:30. I asked everyone that saw me (in a very serious voice) "this doesn't make me look stupid does it? They say this crap is going to make my hair fall out and I don't want to walk out of there bald!!!" Was LOVING the different reactions!!! Couldn't wait to show up at the center...I checked in with the nurse and said the same line.

Nurses were speechless at first....told me "well....you won't lose your hair TODAY"; I said "REALLY? Oh...now I feel stupid!!" After I smiled they roared. She said "honey I'm so happy you came to us, you're going to do just fine".....

5-29-08

Hi Friends...

Not much to report....everything is going extremely well. All weekly blood count checks were normal or better. I'm feeling really good. Thank you for the cards & support, especially your prayers.

I'm not supposed to be thinking about this now… but I can't help it….please pray that I won't need radiation after chemo treatment….it's just something else I hope I won't need.

Next round begins on June 4th I hope the people at the center are ready for me…..I'll be bringing some balloons with me (5 to be exact – one for each treatment I have left); and I'm calling these next sessions my "chemo party". The balloons will be light blue in color. I'm looking forward to talking and praying with others at the center….I will give each balloon away throughout the day to individual patients. I would like to pray with them and would ask them to take a balloon and put all their concerns in there….when they leave that day, I'll ask them to let the balloon go.

I'll let you know how it goes ☺

I'm also writing a book….going to note all of my funny stories and inspirational ideas in it. I'm dedicating the book to God and I really hope it can help people. I hope they would give their troubles over to God, to focus on positives and hopefully it will help them through their struggles.

Until next time…..Thank you for your care, concerns & prayers.
Love,
Kim

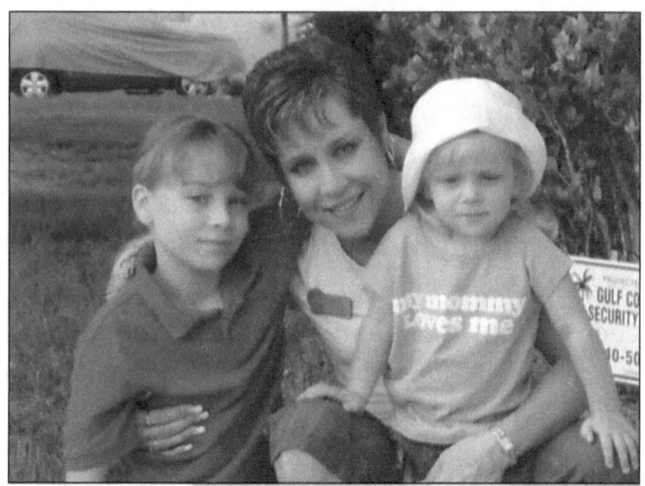

Me and the girls 5-30-08

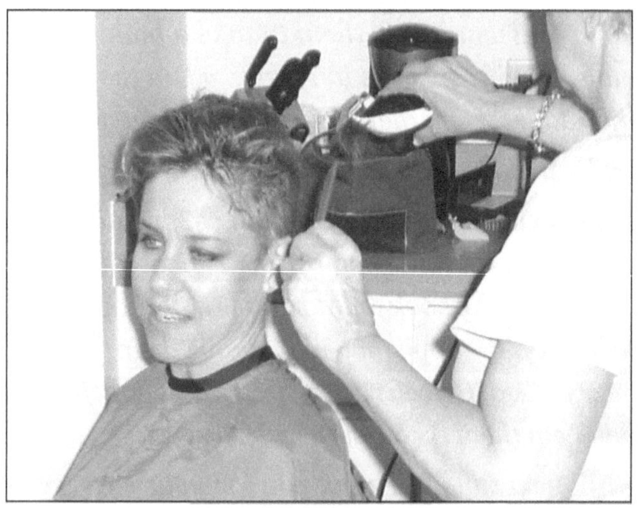

*We (my mom & I) decided I should get a short
hairdo before my hair falls out from treatment.*

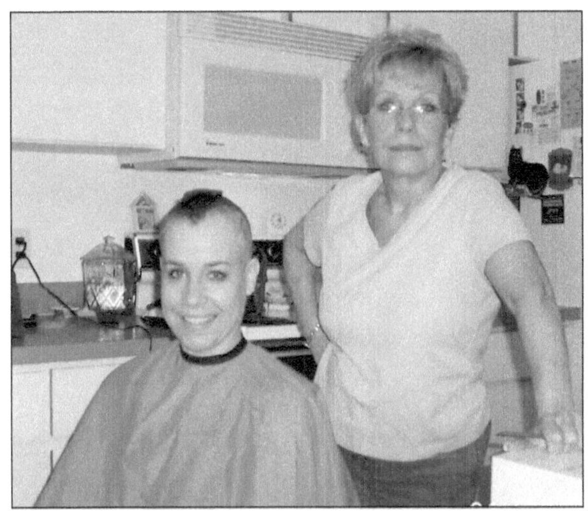

Mohawk for Heather

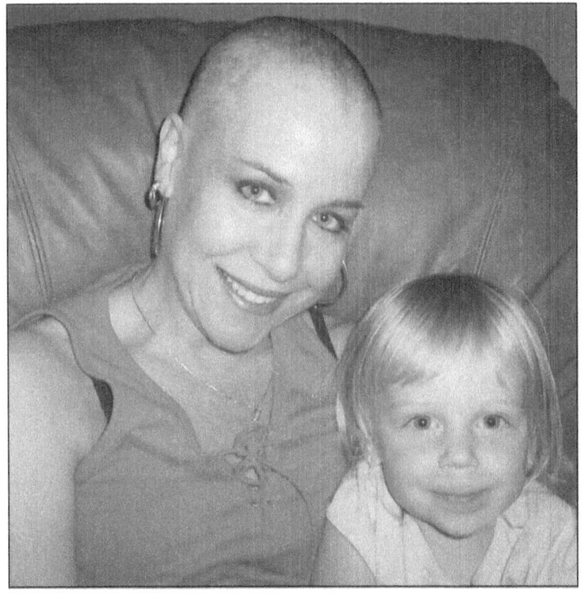

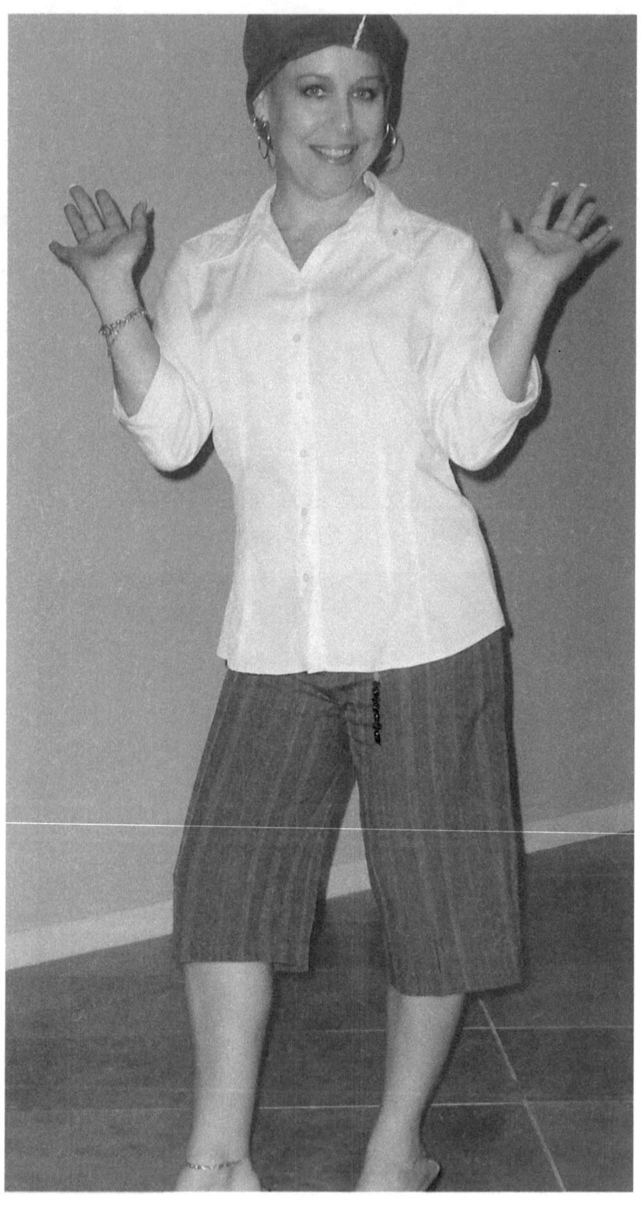

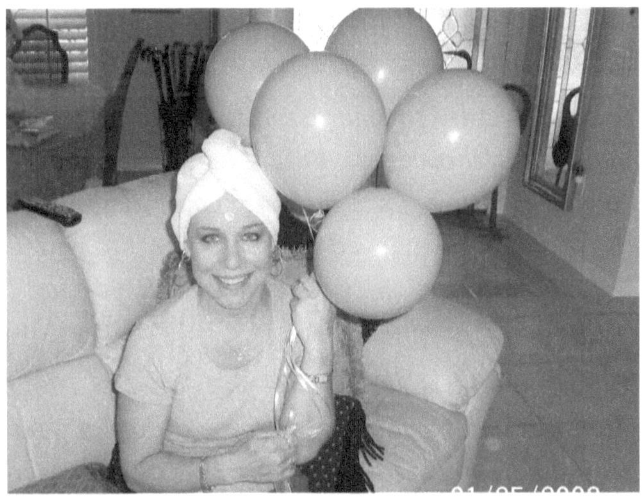

Wed. 6-4-08

Thanks everyone for thinking of me and keeping me in your prayers.

I played a bad joke on Tim this morning. It will go down in Clark history as one of my finest..... he woke late and jumped out of bed. He apologized and told me he couldn't make the kids lunches. I told him not to worry about it I was getting up to prepare things for "my party". As we both scurried around I said while being very busy "Oh can you quickly help me find my curling iron???!?" Without thinking he looks quickly left, looks quickly right, points to a basket where I keep my hair irons and says "Isn't it in that?!?" I just stood very still, very bald & smiling and said "I got you". It took him a couple of seconds and he used the excuse "I'm half asleep!!!"

Today I decided to wear a white turban. It's a lot cooler than those wigs. Before leaving the house I asked Heather if she had any colored stickers. She didn't have any red ones, but she had round yellow "sunshine" stickers....they were perfect! I put it on my forehead.

Anyone who asked me what the dot was, I told them "I thought you had to have a dot on your head when you wear a turban!?!" I told them to just call me "Dottie".

I received a positive report from Dr. Maun, who laughed at my turban & dot and said I need to be there every day; just for his entertainment purposes. He asked if he could come to my office when he is at the club; because he would like to check on me as long as I didn't mind! (I'm thinking??! Heck yeah you can check on me!! How awesome is that?!?). He gave me a big hug and an encouraging look....I feel he is truly wanting me to be well. I'm sure he wants all his patients to get well, but this felt more special in some way.

All went well today and the balloons were a big hit! I told everyone when I walked in that I was glad they were here because they were all invited! Not many people made eye contact or thought I was talking to them.....but I moved on, said hello to everyone I passed and found a chair. I brought a platter of little PB&J sandwiches (as my friend Renee Piney suggested, as some patients forget to eat), also brought a bag of chocolates for the nurses and a specimen cup filled with jelly beans for one nurse (Kelly). She had given me the cup during one visit, but I didn't end up using it. So, when I handed her the cup I told her it took me all week to fill it... just for her and then I popped a jelly bean in my mouth. She was hysterical laughing; then she passed the specimen cup around and everyone gladly took some jelly beans.

Throughout the day I started to tease some of my neighbors (other patients). I told them that they've got to be the most boring party people I have ever met ☺. I said "nobody is dancing, nobody is mingling, everyone just sits there" that got there attention. I pointed to a couple patients that were sleeping and told awake patients "he's not invited to the next party and she's not invited either" HAHAHAHA they all laughed. When the two woke I told them the bad news, then they laughed.

One man (Gene) didn't really participate much in our fun & silliness, at one point I asked my mom to bring him over a balloon and I offered him a sandwich. After that he happily chatted along with the rest of us and he shared his story.

As a few began to leave for the day, they came over to tell me I made their day. One lady (Peggy) said it was the first time she enjoyed a treatment, and she can't wait to see me in 3 weeks. Another guy (Lou) said today was his last treatment, but he'll be stopping by in 3 weeks just to come to the party.

Each had received a balloon with a message that read "Give all your troubles over to God, then let it go". Each came over to hug me and to say good bye, we wished each other the best of luck and I reminded each to be sure and "let it go".

The nurses think I'm nutty, everybody had a smile and it was a really really good day.

One special patient, named Cheryl who is in her 50's I had the opportunity to pray with. She was really the only patient I was strongly compelled to pray with (if she wanted to). I knew of Cheryl having cancer over a year ago. She worked in the dance studio my Heather last attended. She is a single mom with a talented teenage daughter

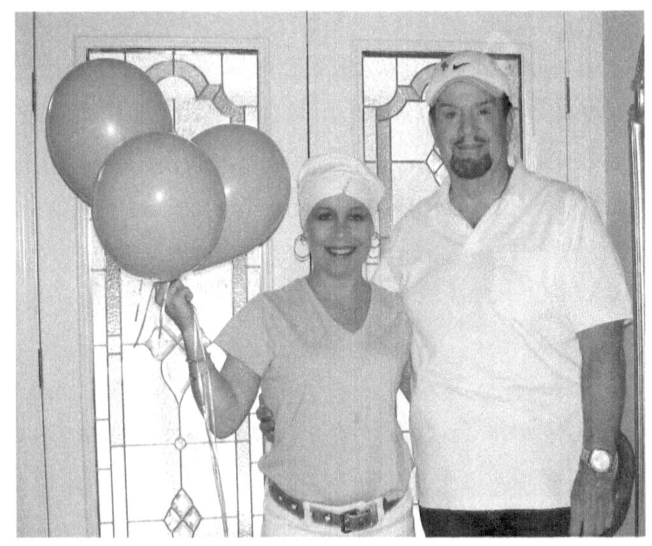

Me with my Dad before treatment

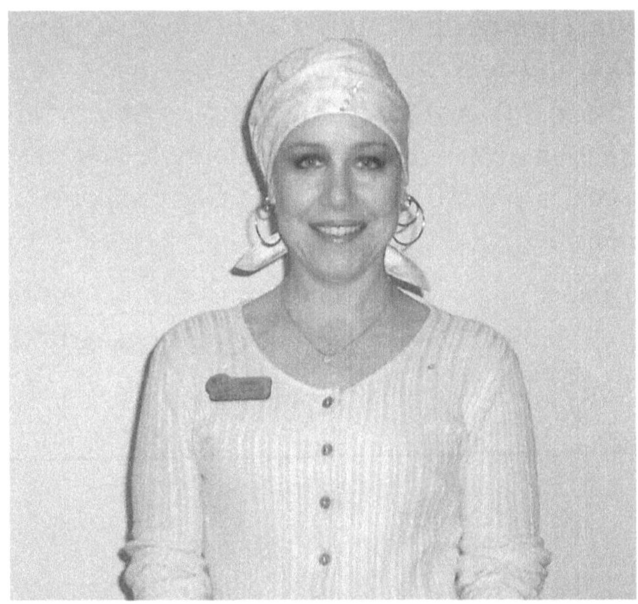

(Sara). Her daughter dances & teaches dance. Sara works at the dance studio where Heather attends now. (A Better Place Dance Studio).

I only recently learned Cheryl has a rare type of lung cancer, she is never expected to be in remission and she will have to have chemotherapy the rest of her life.

I gave her the first balloon with the attached a card. I prayed with her, for her. She had tears and a smile and said she just really needed me today.

I was happy I was able to deliver God's message. I'm looking forward to talking more with her. I'm anxious to tell her what I believe. To me God and only God knows what is in our future. It just isn't something a physician can predict. There may be statistics, there may be educated guesses, but if it is in His plan, God can perform miracles.

Tomorrow will be my actual chemo day....just 2 to 3 hours and I expect it to be fairly uneventful.

Kim

I've given up the wigs....you can't imagine the heat. I'll keep them but only for a wedding or some other event. And I'm donating them when my hair grows but I'm so grateful to Pat (Michele's baby sitter) for hooking me up with these....

I've got solids & prints – something to go with anything....and they feel cool

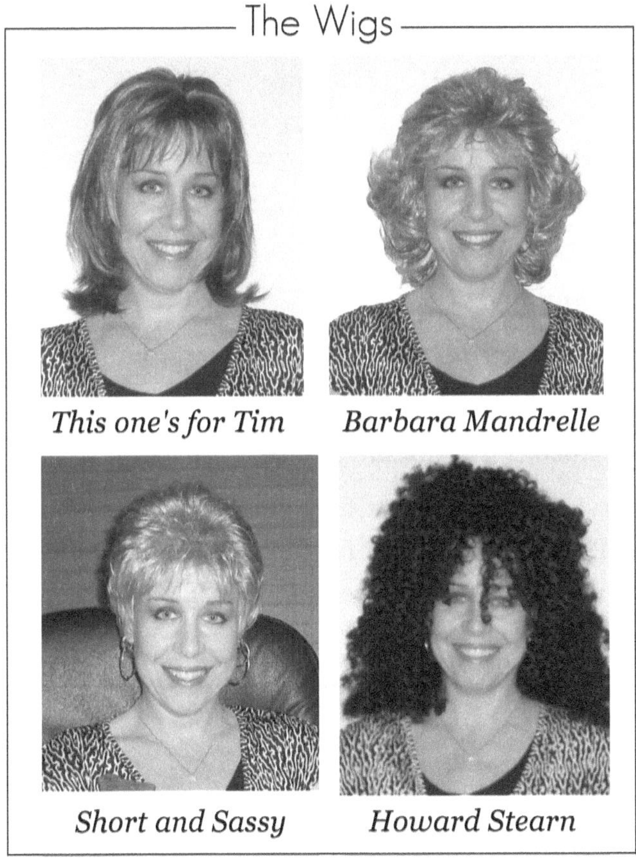

This one's for Tim   *Barbara Mandrelle*

Short and Sassy   *Howard Stearn*

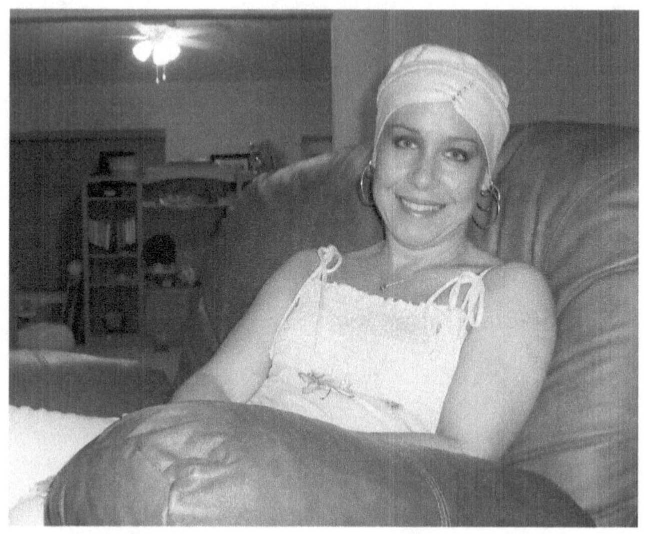

6-29-08

Hi Family & Friends!

3 Down, 3 To Go!

I'm having writer's block – so I'm not sure how humorous this update will be, but I'll give it a go.

First, I should mention what a BIG HELP my DAD has been to us!! He has been with me nearly every treatment; he helps us pick up the kids & takes Heather to camp many mornings. He drives her to Tae Kwon Do. He'll cook meals & bring them over with my mom. Then he patiently sits and watches TV while mom folds clothes, does dishes with me, gives kids baths, has been making new shades for our French doors. — Thanks Dad, you're the best! (After hearing what he said in church...I believe he was feeling a little left out in the cold, so I had to lay it on thick!)

The party on the June 25th didn't seem as eventful as the party on June 4th, but I still brought 4 balloons, chocolates for the nurses/patients & PB&J sandwiches. Mom went with me on day one. We bumped into Gene & Dorothy from treatment 2; I guess we're all becoming regulars. There were still many "sleepers" at the party; I certainly didn't let it go unmentioned.

There were 2 new faces sitting in front of us, a pretty lady (forget her name) and a nice guy named Mike. Both were hooked up to IV's but I couldn't help but notice they HAD HAIR!

I introduced myself to the lady to start up a conversation and boldly asked "So, how come you have hair?" she smiled and said "Oh? I'm not getting chemo, I'm getting iron". I said "Oh really? Iron? Meet me out in the parking lot later, we need to talk". Everybody cracked up. I asked Mike the same thing...."And, you, sir? May I ask how come you have hair?" ...he points his thumb towards the pretty hairy lady and says "I'm like her, I'm just here for iron". I smiled and said, "I guess I'll be meeting you out in the parking lot later as well".

Kelly, the head nurse heard the conversation and yells out "We need security or Kim's going to beat up everybody who has hair". ☺

Well....I didn't let them feel bad.....they each got a balloon! I gave out all 4, with the same note "Give all your troubles over to God, then let it go!"

As people came and went I didn't notice that one balloon was left behind by an older gentle-man.......but just as my treatment was ending, in walked my friend Cheryl! I quickly asked mom to grab the balloon & we gave it to her. I'm sure it was meant for her to have. As soon as I got my IV out, I grabbed Cheryl by the hand and we ran over to a quiet spot to pray. She went with me, as if she knew my plan. I was happy to have the opportunity to pray for her, with her, again.

I give thanks to God, that I feel as well as I feel. I'm beginning to recognize a few side effects, but have remedies to deal with them (dryness in mouth....fatigue hasn't really hit me) I am losing my eyebrows & eyelashes!!! I have a permanent make up client on July 4th so, – I'll probably have my mom tattoo me a few brows too!

Please pray for my friend Renee Piney who,

like Cheryl had lung cancer (except Renee had a lung removed); she is having a complete body scan on July 1st. We're praying that nothing shows up.

I will be regaining strength over the next 2-3 weeks; I will have a CAT scan (chest, neck, abdomen & pelvis) on July 8th. Results may take a week.

My 4th round is July 16th & 17th.
Until next time......

Love,
Kim

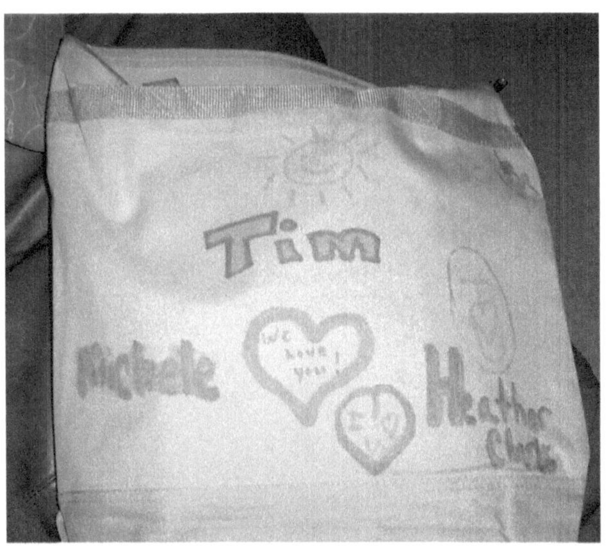

The orange bag

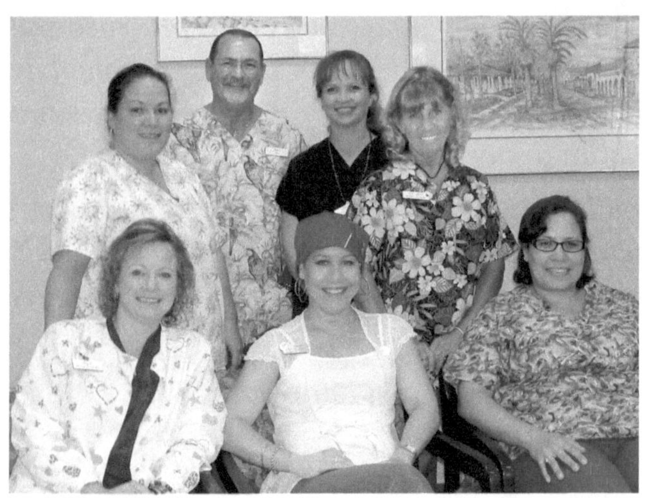

*Back L-R Courtney, Jerry, Teresa, Pat
Front L-R Kelly, Kim, Evette*

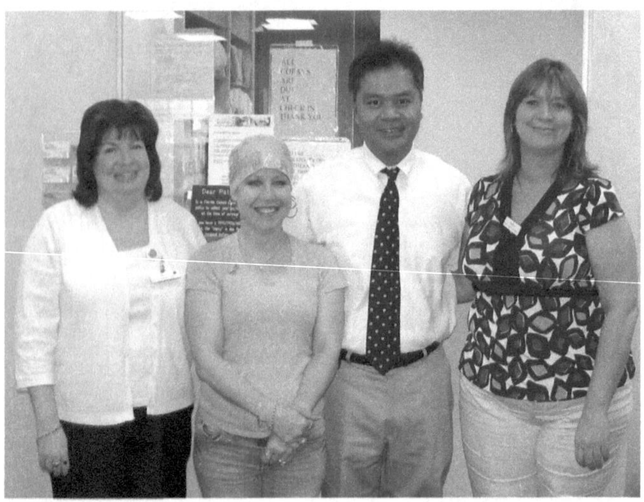

*Me with Beth (left), Nancy (right) and Dr. Maun,
towards the end of chemotherapy treatments.*

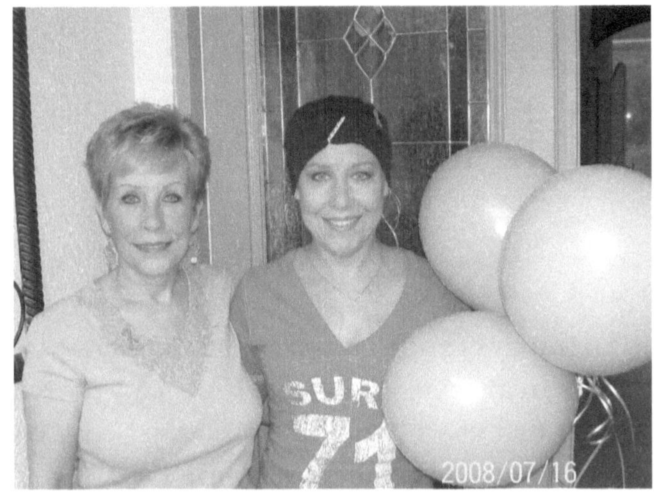

Me with my Mom before treatment 4

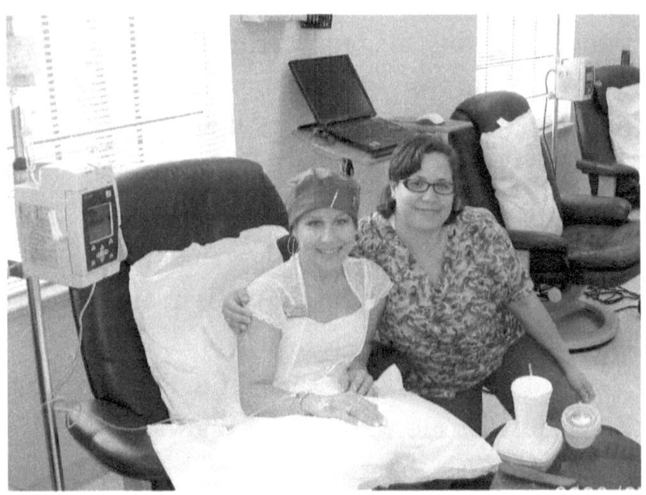

Me with Yvette

CHAPTER 8

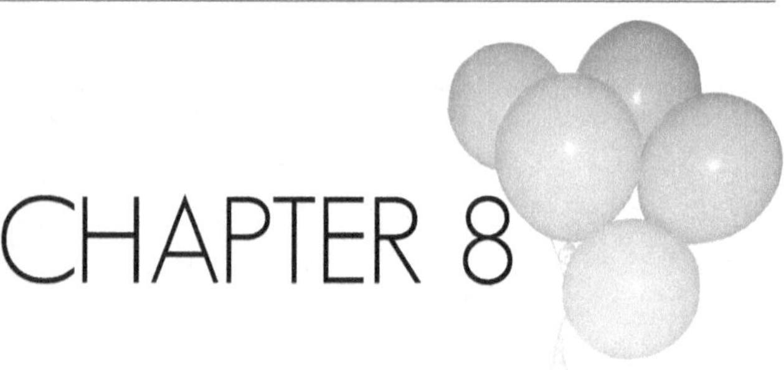

So In July of 2008 I was near the end of my chemo treatments when I suddenly remembered having that chest X-ray at the hospital back on February 2nd, remember back when I was having severe heart burn?

I realized I had never read the X-ray report myself. I realized Dr. Queen had never mentioned receiving the report from the hospital.

Why didn't my doctor mention me going to the hospital or call me for a follow up?

I decided to drive down to the hospital to request a copy of the X-ray. I wondered if the X-ray report had any notations that might have suggested Lymphoma and if those bizarre symptoms had anything to do with Lymphoma.

While I was driving I began to wonder if the ER doctor let me walk out of that hospital with Lymphoma yet told me I had acid reflux. Could they do that? Would they do that?

I pick up the X-ray and as I was reading the

report, I was absolutely beside myself. I couldn't believe what I was reading. It says **"The superior mediastinum is widened and there is a right tracheal soft tissue mass, the heart is not enlarged, the lungs are normal"**.

✸ ✸ ✸

From the time I was diagnosed, I prayed for God to take the lead and I felt God had His hand held out to me, a hand for me to hold as He walked with me. You see, once I was given the diagnosis I was thrown into this whirl-wind almost as if I were in a different dimension. Your mind races with concerns and worries, but other parts of you are put into this assembly line of appointments, meetings, tests and biopsies. It is overwhelming and very, very scary. At first I really didn't make many decisions for myself, as I didn't know what to do or who I should see. I remember praying.

I will never forget the day I was given my diagnosis, it was a Friday afternoon and I was called on my cell while I was at work. I worked at a high-end golf club in Venice. I was the Administrative Assistant. I assisted the General Manager, was responsible for club communications, I was their website administrator, I handled rentals/privileges, estoppels tracking, New member/resident privileges, meeting minutes, receptionist duties, bank deposits, ordered supplies and distributed payroll, just to name a few responsibilities.

The GI specialist asked me where I was and then told me I had Lymphoma. I didn't even know what Lymphoma was. I thought it almost sounds like a cancer, but I didn't know for sure. I had to ask him. Our conversation was short actually – I couldn't think of many questions, I think he gave me instructions for following up with my primary, I really can't remember everything he said after telling me ...."Lymphoma is a blood cancer and you have a large mass above your heart, pressing against your esophagus".

Oh! I did ask if I would need surgery and he said possibly, but more than likely you will have chemotherapy.

I sat there thinking wow, I guess this means I'll be dying soon, and how am I going to tell everyone this? Tim will have to raise our girls alone.... my parents, my poor parents have to see another child die, why Lord? Now, I'm ok with dyeing (I know I'm going to Heaven), I just know how hard it is on the rest of the family. All these things rushing through my head and I still haven't told anyone. I couldn't cry it didn't seem real. What did he say? I didn't ask him how long I have left.

I called Tim on his cell. Man was this hard. I worry enough about him working and driving in difficult weather, but I needed him to pick me up. I wanted to go home and I didn't think I could drive. It broke my heart to give him such news over the phone, he sounded so shaken and said he was coming to get me.

I went over to my co-worker, Simone, and told her Tim was on his way to get me and I needed to go home. After filling her in she hugged me and we held hands.....as I sit here trying to remember all this.....my memory escapes me really, I can only recall pieces. I remember me and Simone going over to our co-worker, Barb, in the golf shop. I told Barb the news and she looked pretty shocked. I remember telling her "I guess God has other plans for me and I have important messages to bring to your loved ones" Barb lost her brother and sister two years ago and then she lost her mom the following year. She and I had many talks about losing family and those talks kept us especially close. Barb replied, "Yeah, but not yet!!!"

Tim arrived to my office in a matter of minutes, he didn't say anything when he saw me, and he just held me.

That night we planned to have dinner at my parent's house. We rounded up the girls and headed over to my mom's house. I was dying inside knowing we were about to break their hearts with the news. My parents remembered I was expecting test results and the first question they asked was "Did the doctor call about your tests? What did they say?" I took mom into her bedroom and sat her down. I left Tim in the kitchen with the kids and my dad and told him to make small talk with dad for a few. When mom and I came out of the room I could tell by my dad's face he was already filled in by Tim. I was mindful of my actions and refused to make this a big dramatic thing. I needed to be strong for them and for my kids. It was however incredibly difficult to eat. We didn't talk much, except to entertain the girls.

Tim and I took the girls home and we privately talked about how we should tell the girls. Michele (2 at the time) wouldn't understand much but Heather (10 at the time) definitely understood something bad was going on, she could tell by everyone's actions at Nanny's house.

I remember taking her and holding her hands and I said "Mommy is sick and I have to have medicine that is so strong it will make my hair fall out in a few weeks, but I didn't mind because the medicine will make me better and then my hair will grow back" She said, "Really?" I said, "Yeah, but you know Nanny is a hair dresser and we're going to have fun and we'll buy some wigs and hats and stuff".

I watched her thinking about what I was telling her and I waited to see if she had any questions. Her next words I will always treasure, she said "oh mommy, if all your hair is going to fall out, then I want to cut my hair off too because I don't want you to be the only one without any hair!" This was the only time I cried. What a precious thing for her to tell me all by herself. Tim and I are constantly correcting Michele's words or filling-in what she means, the same way we taught Heather. Now my big girl is saying this to me. I held her and thanked her and told her "you will NOT cut your hair off young lady".

Another part of sharing a diagnosis is dealing with the different personalities of people. Frankly some reactions were pretty selfish and hurtful; both by friends as well as family.

Mostly everyone in our lives were wonderful to us, our employers and immediate families were so warm, loving, supportive and gracious.

Tim and I spent many weekends going to dinner with another family; we even spent one weekend together in Orlando. They find out I have cancer, and we never see them again. Not a note, not a call. Nothing. That hurt. I would never have done that to them if the tables were turned. My parents were right when I was a kid they told me many times; keep your faith in God not in people.

Your friends will disappoint you.

There were similar reactions from my own family! .....I was just surprised by the reactions from people or the lack of reactions I should say. I was going through a tough situation. They didn't feel it was necessary to communicate. That's not how I would have treated them, but? Hey! I'll save a few dollars on Christmas cards.

Unfortunately I've met many people with cancer. I've worked with several people with cancer. I was especially touched by a brave woman named Nancy when I worked at Prestanica from 2001 to 2004. She was diagnosed with breast cancer and I remember being so hurt that such a kind, likable lady would have to endure something so difficult. I remember telling her how easily her diagnosis could have been mine (meaning, any woman). I've always felt extremely vunerable to breast cancer. I watch the news and hear the statistics, and have dealt with cancer in my immediate family. I felt a need to show her intimate support. A group of us had a luncheon for her as a send off before she began her treatment. I really didn't do much, but I did what I could. I would pray for her, I would call to check on her, I sent her encouraging cards and I would remind her she was missed at work (and she was). I followed the "golden rule".

How would I feel if I were the one having to go through that? After all, this could have been me! And guess what? One day it was me.

✸ ✸ ✸

I had worked at a golf club in Venice with a girl, Lori Ann, who battled Sarcoma the entire time I worked with her. I even took her to a couple of her chemo appointments! She and I became friends. The day I was diagnosed, she was one of the calls I made. I remember telling her, "Well, my friend, it seems that we're both in the battle, I was diagnosed today with Lymphoma." She was positively crushed by my news, but in a weird way it was of some comfort to me knowing someone else with cancer – at work—in my real world. So, when I was told who my Oncologist was going to be, I called Lori Ann. I said to her "so, I know who my Oncologist is. Have you heard of a Dr. Maun, Noel Maun?" She hesitates, thinking I was joking and says, "Kim, are you serious? Dr. Maun is a member of our club, you set up his privileges!"

After we hung up, I walked over to the golf shop and asked Barb if she knows Dr. Maun, I explained that he's my new Oncologist Barb looks down at the tee sheet and says, "Yep, Dr. Maun is just about to the 9th hole." I was flabbergasted!

Here I was about to enter this insane world of cancer treatments and the very person going to care for me is not only a member where I work, but he is playing golf right outside my office. You can't tell me that isn't God's hand.

Dr. Maun is with Florida Cancer Specialists in Venice and he and his staff are tops! Thank you Dr. Maun, you're the best.

After I completed chemotherapy, Dr. Maun wanted me to meet the radiologist to discuss radiation therapy. I was still hoping they would determine I didn't need radiation. I was not looking forward to having these treatments whatsoever. The radiologist was very informative and honest. He thoroughly explained the procedure and why radiation was necessary. I brought a list of questions and he answered them.

The radiologist explained the radiation would be "very unpleasant." The reason had to do with the location that had to be focused on, they needed to radiate my neck, chest, breast and underarm areas. All the places the tumor was and places where cells could be hiding. It was crucial to zap all areas where cells could linger or they could grow. He said the radiation would cause me to have an extremely sore throat—oh, how I hate sore throats! I asked, "How sore?" He said it would probably feel like the worst sore throat you have ever had. This would last for two weeks and I could expect soreness for two additional weeks after treatment while the area healed on the inside. I would be on a liquid diet, so I should expect to lose weight. If I was not able to get the liquids down, they would need to give me a feeding tube. In the next few weeks (before treatments begins), I am able to eat whatever I want – no diet restrictions, the more weight I gain, the better it will be for me. In addition, the treatments themselves wouldn't be a picnic either, as they would have to place me in a very awkward and uncomfortable position. He said they would have my arms up above my head and my neck would be tilted up and as far back as it could possibly go, and then they will tilt it back even further. I would have to lie perfectly still in this position for 20 minutes and I cannot move a muscle, every day 5 days per week. (Not sure how many treatments, but it would be somewhere around 20 to 30). And finally, the future risks of radiation—I thought to myself, 'Does this doctor have any good news?' with radiation to my chest/neck comes additional risks (future risks) of breast cancer, potential heart complications, trouble swallowing, throat cancer, etc.

He gave us the date he would like me to begin treatment and we left.

I was overwhelmed and extremely worried and so I prayed. We all prayed.

I still wanted to know more—more like a second opinion, but who? There was so much for me to think about, on top of working, taking care of our home, husband & two kids.

So, one day I'm reading the mail and noticed a flyer from the National Leukemia & Lymphoma Society. World-renowned lymphoma specialist Dr. Zelenetz will lead September teleconference. I took note of the date and planned to participate as it was just what I needed! How neat to be able to speak directly to a world-renowned lymphoma specialist! I could ask him all my questions about radiation and get his opinion.

The date of the teleconference came and went before I knew it. Two days after it had already taken place, I decided to check to see when it was. I was so disappointed that I missed it. As a matter of fact, I was beside myself! I was so mad at myself I couldn't stop thinking about missing this opportunity!

I decided to call the hospital in New York where the specialist works. Little did I know at the time that he practiced in one of the world's leading hospitals for cancer and cancer research, if not it's the world's leading cancer hospital, Memorial Sloan Kettering Cancer Center. I figured I would tell his office that I missed the teleconference, I'm a lymphoma patient and I really had some important questions. Almost as if his assistant expected the next words out of my mouth, she said "Fax me your records and your questions; I'll have Dr. Z. review your records and he'll give you a determination." I thought to myself, "He will? Really?" I was so excited.

A couple of days later, I called his office to check and see if they received my fax. Like I was right around the corner, his assistant said, "Dr. Z. has reviewed your files and he wants to see you. Can you come in on Thursday?" I was numb with surprise; this world-renowned specialist wants to see ME? But I coolly replied, "Yes, yes I can see him Thursday. What time?" *I'm thinking HELLO? I live in FLORIDA!* She gives me the time and we hang up. I was so scared and excited at the same time and was thinking *how am I going to get a ticket and go to NY?*

I couldn't dial my mom and talk fast enough. I explain: the flyer, world-renowned, wants to see me, he's in NY, an extremely prestigious facility, and I have an appointment with him on Thursday!! My mom was so happy for me. She said, "Don't worry about a thing! I'm going with you! I'll have Dad call your Aunt Mame and Aunt Bea!" (They live in NY).

I'm thinking, "I guess we're going to NY on Thursday" (like it's a ride around the block.) How funny is this!? If you haven't already guessed, I don't travel much and I can count on one hand how many times I've flown.

That afternoon my mom just about had everything planned and arranged. She said my dad had the tickets. My Aunt Mame (Mary Castellano) and her husband Vito (Ret. General Vito Castellano) would pick us up at JFK, bring us to their beach house, take us to my appointment and back to the airport. It was, in fact, as simple as pie. I have no doubt that God made these arrangements and all the pieces fell right into place. It was just so neat. You can't tell me that isn't God's hand.

Another e-mail:

9-28-08

Dear Friends & Family,

Hi! I'm SO HAPPY to be on the ground. I felt like kissing the pavement when we landed in Tampa. By now most of you know I don't travel often and have only flown twice before.

A little humor about the trip back.....my mom and I were comfortably sitting in the terminal at JFK unknowingly at the wrong gate for nearly an hour. We ate, we talked, we were so confident being where we were. I kept checking my ticket which said "Gate 26 SEP"....we were to depart at 12:55 and the time was 12:50 but nobody was on line to go on the plane. So? I glance back at the ticket and now realized it said "Date 26 SEP". I freaked out and ran to a nearby gate and asked a Delta pilot "Where does this thing list the gate?! Our plane is about to take off!!" Needless to say, my mom and I went from a calm & comfortable mode to complete havoc....which included the famous O.J. Simpson sprint across the airport to GATE 20 (but we didn't look nearly as graceful by any means....both of us with a bag in each arm running like mad women)....just embarrassing to say the least.

The visit with Dr. Z. was fantastic. Everything from our trip up, the assistance from my Aunt Mame & Vito...and back, everything was seamless.

The minute I stepped foot into Sloan center I could just "feel the knowledge & experience"....

To sum up a nearly 2 hour meeting, Dr. Z. does recommend that I have radiation. He recommended a specific strength "30-grey" of which he will send to my oncologist & treating radiologist in FL. He answered each and every question I brought with me, but did so with explanation and support. They were not rushed or impatient. I left there with a better understanding and another supportive prognosis.

He went over the potential risks that the first radiologist mentioned, but he gave us his opinion about them (i.e. potential for heart complications and/or breast cancer in the future). For the most part he feels there is "potential" for this in the future, but I understood his feeling about them doesn't deserve a lot of focus. Potential doesn't mean it WILL happen it COULD happen. He explained the risks of potential breast cancer like this....if I were in my 20's the radiation would increase my chances 10-15%. But, at my age the radiation wouldn't increase my chances any more than any other woman on the street.

He went over the scary radiation side effects and again, his feeling about them seemed to have less prevalence. The sore throat & difficulty swallowing will be tolerable....he doesn't think I'll require a feeding tube, etc. Everything didn't seem to be as bad according to Dr. Z. It was relieving news.

He showed us where the mass was on the X-ray taken on 2/2/08, and he even drew a diagram to help us understand what the reduction in the mass looked like and potentially where it would be now. It's basically in an area that is undetectable by any equipment they have today.....so judging from past cases they found that radiation significantly reduces the potential of reoccurrence.

There was a lot more discussed, but for now you've got the picture. I anticipate starting radiation in the next few days, I'll keep you posted.

My mom and I are extremely grateful to Aunt Mame and Vito for all their help and hospitality. Thank you both so much!! You made an extremely tense situation feel like a happy reunion and a lovely visit. Your beach house is so sweet and cozy. Your love is immeasurable. Thank you for going with me Mame. Vito's patience is unheard of.

And...it was a nice surprise to see Michael!! (NY cousin). Thanks for driving down Mike.

This entire trip from beginning to end was absolutely guided by God's hand, and that is evident to me and my family by all of the things that happened and how they happened. I simply cannot recall them all, but it was practically a moment to moment occurrence, from the things we did, to the feelings & assurances we received. When this started, I asked the Lord to take control, and that He has.

Thank you for keeping us in your prayers.

With love and thanks,
Kim & family

During spring 2008 my friend & co-worker Lori Ann wasn't doing well with her treatments and her prognosis looked grim. I had just begun my Lymphoma battle but she had been fighting Sarcoma going on 5 years. I was thinking of ways I could be an encouragement to her when I remembered a beautiful e-mail forward and I used the message in a neat way. First here is the forward: (Thank you April for sending me this).

The Thorns

This is a bit long, but really worth the read...

Sandra felt as low as the heels of her shoes when she pulled open the florist shop door, against a November gust of wind. Her life had been as sweet as a spring breeze and then, in the fourth month of her second pregnancy, a "minor" automobile accident stole her joy. This was Thanksgiving week and the time she should have delivered their infant son. She grieved over their loss. Troubles had multiplied.

Her husband's company "threatened" to transfer his job to a new location. Her sister had called to say that she could not come for her long awaited holiday visit. What's worse, Sandra's friend suggested that Sandra's grief was a God-given path to maturity that would allow her to empathize with others who suffer. "She has no idea what I'm feeling," thought Sandra with a shudder. "Thanksgiving? Thankful for what?" she wondered. "For a careless driver whose truck was hardly scratched when he rear-ended her? For an airbag that saved her life, but took her child's?"

"Good afternoon, can I help you?"

Sandra was startled by the approach of the shop clerk. "I . . . I need an arrangement," stammered Sandra.

"For Thanksgiving? I'm convinced that flowers tell stories," she continued. "Are you looking for something that conveys 'gratitude' this Thanksgiving?"

"Not exactly!" Sandra blurted out. "In the last five months, everything that could go wrong has gone wrong."

Sandra regretted her outburst, and was surprised when the clerk said, "I have the perfect arrangement for you."

Then the bell on the door rang, and the clerk greeted the new customer, "Hi, Barbara, let me get your order." She excused herself and walked back to a small workroom, then quickly reappeared, carrying an arrangement of greenery, bows, and what appeared to be long-stemmed thorny roses. Except the ends of the rose stems were neatly snipped; there were no flowers.

"Do you want these in a box?" asked the clerk. Sandra watched "was this a joke? Who would want rose stems with no flowers! She waited for laughter, but neither woman laughed.

"Yes, please," Barbara replied with an appreciative smile. "You'd think after three years of getting the special, I wouldn't be so moved by its significance, but I can feel it right here, all over again," she said, as she gently tapped her chest.

Sandra stammered, "Ah, that lady just left with . . . uh . . . she left with no flowers!"

"That's right, said the clerk." I cut off the flowers. That's the 'Special'. I call it the Thanksgiving Thorns Bouquet. Barbara came into the shop three years ago, feeling much as you do today," explained the clerk. "She thought she had very little to be thankful for. She had just lost her father to cancer; the family business was failing; her son had gotten into drugs; and she was facing major surgery. That same year I had lost my husband," continued the clerk. "For the first time in my life, I had to spend the holidays alone. I had no children, no husband, no family nearby, and too much debt to allow any travel."

"So what did you do?" asked Sandra.

"I learned to be thankful for thorns," answered the clerk quietly. "I've always thanked God for the good things in my life and I never questioned Him why those good things happened to me, but when the bad stuff hit, I cried out, Why? Why me? It took time for me to learn that the dark times are important to our faith! I have always enjoyed the 'flowers' of my life, but it took the thorns to show me the beauty of God's comfort! You know, the Bible says that God comforts us when we're afflicted, and from His consolation we learn to comfort others."

Sandra sucked in her breath, as she thought about what her friend had tried to tell her. "I guess the truth is I don't want comfort. I've lost a baby and I am angry with God."

Just then someone else walked in the shop.

"Hey, Phil!" the clerk greeted the balding, rotund man.

"My wife sent me in to get our usual

Thanksgiving arrangement . . . twelve thorny, long-stemmed stems!" laughed Phil as the clerk handed him a tissue wrapped arrangement from the refrigerator.

"Those are for your wife?" asked Sandra incredulously. "Do you mind telling me why she wants a bouquet that looks like that?"

"Four years ago, my wife and I nearly divorced," Phil replied. "After forty years, we were in a real mess, but with the Lord's grace and guidance, we trudged through problem after problem, the Lord rescued our marriage. Jenny here (the clerk) told me she kept a vase of rose stems to remind her of what she had learned from "thorny" times. That was good enough for me. I took home some of those stems. My wife and I decided to label each one for a specific "problem" and give thanks for what that problem taught us."

As Phil paid the clerk, he said to Sandra, "I highly recommend the Special!"

"I don't know if I can be thankful for the thorns in my life" Sandra said to the clerk. "It's all too . . fresh."

"Well," the clerk replied carefully, "my experience has shown me that the thorns make the roses more precious. We treasure God's providential care more during trouble than at any other time. Remember that it was a crown of thorns that Jesus wore so we might know His love. Don't resent the thorns."

Tears rolled down Sandra's cheeks. For the first time since the accident, she loosened her grip on her resentment.

"I'll take those twelve long-stemmed thorns, please," she managed to choke out.

"I hoped you would," said the clerk gently. "I'll have them ready in a minute."

"Thank you. What do I owe you?"

"Nothing. Nothing but a promise to allow God to heal your heart. The first year's arrangement is always on me."

The clerk smiled and handed a card to Sandra. "I'll attach this card to your arrangement, but maybe you would like to read it first."

It read:

"My God, I have never thanked You for my thorns. I have thanked You a thousand times for my roses, but never once for my thorns. Teach me the glory of the cross I bear; teach me the value of my thorns. Show me that I have climbed closer to You along the path of pain. Show me that, through my tears, the colors of Your rainbow look much more brilliant."

Praise Him for the roses; thank Him for the thorns.

God Bless all of you. Be thankful for all that the Lord does for you.

"Live simply, love generously, care deeply, speak kindly, and leave the rest to God."

Isn't that a special message? Anyway I decided to contact a florist we used at the club (Addington's Florist); the owner had known Lori Ann for several years. I asked if they would give me some rose stems. When I told her my idea & that it was for Lori Ann, they not only gave me the rose stems, they gave me the boxes and bows too!

I printed the e-mail story in booklet form and I personalized each, I attached the booklet to the box of rose stems & dressed them with the bow.

I gave one to my mom (it was near anniversary 9 of my brother Sean's passing).

I gave one to my friend/co-worker Barb, she lost her brother and sister two years before; two days apart, her brother died Christmas Eve & her sister died two days later. She then lost her mom the following year in November.

I brought the third one to Lori Ann, her health was declining.

I enjoyed leaving everyone the boxes, but more importantly was the message.

Sadly, Lori Ann passed away.

Remembering a special lady
Lori Ann Reid lost her battle with
Sarcoma May 22, 2008

Remember in Chapter 4 I talked about the "forever kisses"? While having lunch one day with Lori Ann I told her I gathered kisses from my brother Sean prior to his passing and how I gave my family the boxes. She told me she absolutely loved the idea. We had a very in depth conversation about life & death. How uncertain things are, etc. We were both very candid with each other, so it didn't feel inappropriate for me to simply ask "would that be something you would want to do, leave kisses to your family? I could help do that if you wanted me to?" She said "definitely".

So, from time to time I would remind her to get me a list of names and addresses. I wanted her to write me a list while she was well enough. And one day she did gave me a small list. Lori Ann's health rapidly declined.

When her husband called me to tell me the doctor's had only given Lori Ann two days at the most to live, the first thing that came to my mind was fulfilling her request.

I asked him if he would do me a favor, but please don't ask any questions. He agreed. I asked him to get a plastic bag and bring it to Lori Ann and just say "blow some kisses into this bag for me". He said he would. I told him she would know what it was for.

When he called to tell me of Lori Ann's passing, I asked him if he got the kisses? He said he did and that Lori Ann said there were a couple of hugs in there too. It made me smile.

I made arrangements to pick up the bag of kisses a few days before her funeral and I put together the boxes and personalized them according to her list.

Inside her husband, Bill and only daughter, Jessica's box each also had a yellow ribbon. I explained in their card that the ribbon was for when they wanted a hug from Lori Ann, they just had to wrap the ribbon around your shoulders and hold it tight.

I used a yellow ribbon because that was Lori Ann's favorite color.

Several days later I received warm messages from her loved ones and her closest friend. Not only were they touched by the gesture, the fact that they were truly filled with kisses from her makes them a treasure. Everyone felt it was the neatest idea. I'm happy I was able to help give another family forever kisses from their loved one.

CHAPTER 9

learned important lessons. To be more of my own doctor, always get copies of test results and read them! I'm grateful I spoke up and demanded the scan; my doctor was complacent and negligent. I will continue to "listen to that voice" that sense (feeling) God has given us when something doesn't seem right. I ask lots of questions.

I never felt that God gave me cancer or that I was being punished. I actually felt that my diagnosis and going through treatments wasn't about me at all. If my hunch is correct, then I feel honored that the Lord used me in that way. I told several people that I had a feeling God might have been trying to reach people around me, perhaps by the way I handled the hardship or by my giving it over to God.

In Oct. 2008 I broke up with our doctor. I needed to see him in person (my dad came with me) and I read him the complaint letter I wrote to his Chief Medical Officer. I needed him to know how I felt, he ignored my symptoms and that cost me between 3 & 4 months lead time on my diagnosis and treatments. After all, the cancer motto is practically "early diagnosis, early treatments" right? "Get tested....find it early"?

Anyway, he seemed sorrowful and he apologized, I hugged him and although it was difficult I forgave him.

I was advised to file complaints with the AHCA & Department of Health on both the doctor and also the hospital and I did so. The hospital failed to tell me what the x-ray report said and/or they failed to notify my physician. They let me walk out of their facility twice without notifying me (or my doctor) the findings on the x-ray report (Feb. 2nd and again on Apr. 17th).

Not one person, not a physician or administrative personnel at either facility took ownership of these grievous errors. Not one person offered to help us out in any way. No gestures. I suppose if someone there had given us money to help with the never ending co-pays & medical bills; it would have been an admission of guilt. So instead they do nothing for a family they treated for over 10 years. This obviously seemed appropriate to him. A reputation is worth so much more than your patient's live. Thanks "Doc".

Nothing monetary came from this; everybody

pointed the finger at each other. Everyone said they were sorry, but nobody was at fault.

Basically I was told "since you are alive, you have no case". If either the physician or the hospital had given me the exact treatment and I had fallen into a coma, had left the facility missing a body part or if I had died, I would have had a solid case.

Simply stated, physicians and hospitals can treat you any way they want to and get away with it. They don't have to give you anything and they won't.

My life is worth nothing (money value) to someone not related to me. They can and will let you walk away with a serious disease, you can prove they did this and it will be proven to not be their fault. Someone at one point even said "Well? They didn't give you cancer".

The good news is I am priceless in God's eyes. I'm priceless in my kid's eyes, my husband's eyes. I'm grateful to have survived and it looks like I will see my girls grow up.

We are only here for a season and I look forward to my rewards in Heaven. I may have medical bills, but I'm blessed.

Proverbs 3:5-6 Trust in the Lord with all your heart, and lean not on your own understanding; in all your ways acknowledge him, and he will make your paths straight.

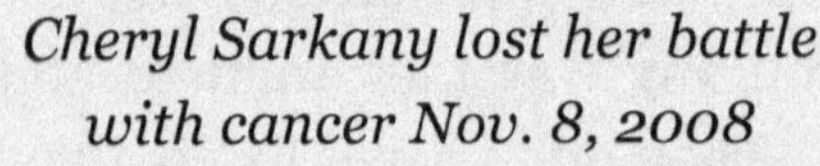

Remembering two special ladies.
I went through treatments with them
and prayed with them:

Cheryl Sarkany lost her battle
with cancer Nov. 8, 2008

Dorothy Hart lost her battle
with cancer Dec. 19, 2008

CHAPTER 10

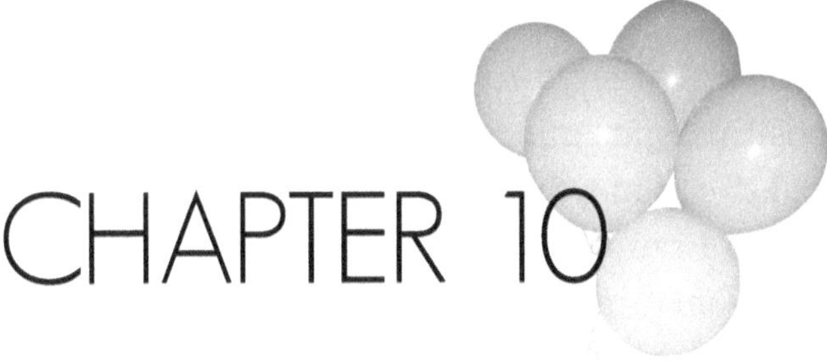

One morning in early October 2009 I was on my way to an interview. It felt good to be going on an interview. By this time I had been laid off nearly 6 months. So I was more than eager to interview. I left the house nearly an hour before I needed to, to give myself time to run an errand and have some lunch. I wanted to return a blouse at Bealls and I figured I would buy myself lunch with the money from returning the blouse. We stopped eating out weeks ago, so I thought of going to lunch as a reward for trying (to find a job).

You might think I'm crazy for saying this, but I think I handled being diagnosed with Lymphoma better than I handled being laid off from that job. My husband might even agree with me.

While on the drive I began thinking about how badly I needed a job, but I wanted another good job. I wasn't sure what to expect on this interview so I prayed. I began to compile in my mind the financial situation we were in and I began to worry myself. I wanted to go to this interview with a positive, open mind but the emotional and financial situation we were in dominated my thoughts.

So I ran into Bealls to return the blouse and the woman at the desk spoke broken English. She is explaining to me that she can only give me store credit since I didn't have a receipt. I explained that I don't normally shop there, I was on my way to an appointment and I really just wanted my money back, could she please make an exception? While the woman goes to check with her supervisor and I wait for the judges ruling; I get this sudden hot wave of emotions come over me and I begin to softly cry. It was absolutely uncontrollable. The more I fought back the emotions, the more I seemed to cry. I'm doing my best to keep my composure and I began thinking I should just walk out, leave the blouse altogether when the supervisor arrived. I gain enough composure to explain that I didn't want a store credit, would she mind giving me the money back. Maybe the supervisor picked up my emotions I don't know, but she didn't speak, she just handed me the refund. I thank her for her time, and I begin to collect my things and as I was putting the cash away it was the supervisor who touched me on my shoulder and said "Better things are yet to come".

❋ ❋ ❋

This was where I started the book....

Now I was on my way to meet the Executive Director, Dan Dunn of All Faiths Food Bank located in Sarasota. He and I met at a restaurant in Venice for the interview. I remember praying for the interview to go well, even if I wasn't offered the position. It just felt good being considered for any position with the economy being the way it has been. I knew so many people in the same situation. Times are very tough.

Before I continue I have to add something cute that happened the day Dan called me for the interview. I got up early to check my e-mail and to see if there were any new positions. I immediately e-mailed my resume to two businesses, one needing an office manager and the other needing an executive assistant. I left my computer and began to make my bed when the phone rings. It was Dan Dunn. He said he was calling in reference to my resume. The first thing I said to him was "You're kidding, I just hit send!" We laughed and went back and forth a little about e-mail etiquette in a light hearted way I said you're not supposed to read the last e-mail that comes in first, you should always scroll to the top. He said he never does that, he saw mine first and so he called.

Dan was professional and extremely knowledgeable about the organization. He had a much laid back personality and was extremely pleasant. He asked questions about my experience and education and he described the position he had open. I immediately knew I could handle the job, I was positive I would be ideal for the position and the position would be ideal for me. I wondered if the environment was as pleasant as the golf club, but it was not my main concern.

When the interview was over he explained he had other people to interview but we remained he would call me in a day or two. He had planned to make a decision for the position very soon.

I had such a good feeling when I got home, but I didn't want my hopes to be premature. I remember praying if it was God's will I could really use this job. And now that I met Dan and felt positive feelings; I really wanted it.

The next morning Dan called to invite me to the food bank to tour the facility. I was kind of nervous, but anxious to see everything. I was surprised with the facility and I was extremely impressed by what they are able to accomplish. The building is pretty new and it has 2 stories; the top floor is the executive offices, board room with a kitchen area and a small event room. The bottom part is an enormous warehouse, big sorting room, a store, a huge walk-in refrigeration/freezer, a break room and it's very busy.

Once we were finished with the tour we discussed more about the position. To my surprise he offered me the job! It was an answer to our prayers. After 6 months of unemployment and all the stresses that come from it, I was so happy and thankful to be back to work! I later find out the food bank received between 250 – 277 resumes for my position. My resume was the one Dan saw first? I believe God had His hand in this and I'm so grateful.

I was given an opportunity to help the needy in our community. I went from serving 25 years in the corporate business world into nonprofit and it is like night and day. The staff here likes their jobs. There are only 21 paid positions. They have over 300 volunteers.

This nonprofit organization is extremely well run and respected and my job is very rewarding in so many ways. I am doing things I've never done; I'm being educated in public speaking as well as grant writing. I attend the finest functions with some of the most prominent and influential people in our community (including senators, congressmen and philanthropists). We're in the paper all the time and the girls at work know I get the biggest kick out of seeing my picture/name in the paper. I'm teased because I keep a file of my newspaper photos; I call it my "file of fame". So now when we expect the local news stations to be around, the girls watch my reactions; they get a kick out of me trying to get into the shot. (I've even been paged "Kim ABC-7 is here!")

Now, one day I was actually interviewed while attending our annual letter carriers food drive! Everybody said I did a nice job, but to be honest I was so nervous! But yay! I was on TV!

Besides being the Executive Director's Assistant, I handle a lot of our Marketing. I do most of the graphics (designing posters, flyers, brochures, announcements, press releases and magazine publications) for our events and some of our programs. I assist with and attend the events (many times with my family), I respond to the e-mails from our website; I take meeting minutes, I organize capital campaign luncheons and take people on tours, and I help lead people in the community to our partner agencies for assistance. People who have been laid off from their job, like I was. People who have never found themselves in this vulnerable position and their need to ask for assistance. We help children, adults and the elderly with dignity and respect.

And since I know he'll be reading my book, I would like Mr. Dunn to know how much I love and appreciate my job. I greatly respect him. He is an awesome leader. Thank you Dan. Should I ask for next Friday off now or should I send you an e-mail?☺

CHAPTER 11

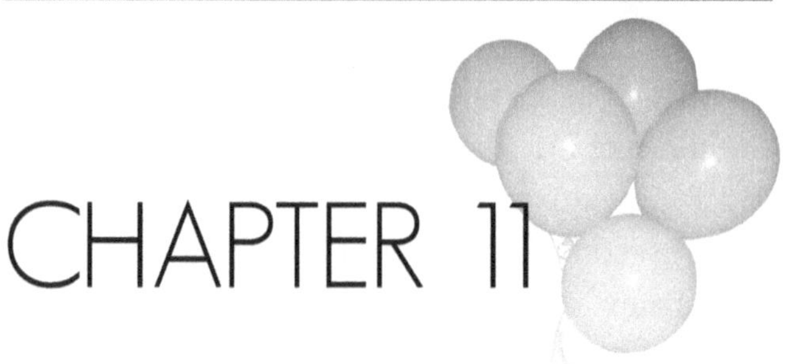

There is another special friend I had been praying for. She had been battling ovarian cancer the last 3 years. Her name is Jare Whitmore (pronounced Jerry).

We attended the same church for many years and eventually both our families stopped attending that church, but she and I remained close through e-mails and phone calls. We had more than just church in common.

I referred her to my Oncologist, Dr. Maun and she did see him over the last several months. Her cancer was advanced, she underwent several surgeries and she had already received a few different rounds of treatments. She was not responding as they would have hoped.

Eventually Jare would not be receiving any further treatments and the family was advised to consider a hospice facility for her care. I went to visit her in October 2010 she was doing remarkably well and she wasn't in any pain. She and her husband were thoroughly impressed with her care.

I planned to discuss the "forever kisses" with her to see if she liked the idea. They had recently had a family reunion (they have tons of grand kids) and that's when the thought occurred to me. Will I get to do this again?

I came across a bunch of cute little boxes in the event room at the food bank, gift card boxes. I put about 20 of them into a bag and kept the bag in my truck.

Just before Thanksgiving 2010 I learned Jare's health was rapidly declining. I still needed to see if she liked the idea of the kisses. Plus I was preparing for our annual family trip for the holiday.

I happened to be running Food Bank errands just off Clark Road (which is close to the hospice facility) and so I swing in to see her, and I brought the bag of boxes.

She was resting and was a little out of it but she welcomed my surprise visit.

I tell her about the boxes of kisses I collected from Sean and how I collected Lori Ann's kisses for her family. Jare loved the idea. I told her I thought she would and so I came prepared and I pulled out the bag of boxes, I held the bag open and she blew kisses and I caught them.

I got out a pen and she carefully went through each of her kid's names and each of their kids names. 18 names, plus her husband, sister and brother.

We prayed before I left. I drove home with mixed feelings. Sadness – she was dying and that would probably be the last time I would see her (on earth). Gratefulness – her pain would soon be over. Wonder – why I recovered and she, Lori Ann, Cheryl and others I know did not.

I was uncomfortable putting the boxes together that night, but I was leaving for our trip and they only gave Jare a couple of days. And I wanted her family to have her kisses, and she was counting on me.

I really have doing these boxes down pat. I prepared labels with all the names, labels with "forever kisses", labels with "Open when you need a kiss from Jare (some said Mom & a bunch said Nana).

It's my third group of forever kisses and I get to give them to her loved ones! How neat is that? Once I put them together I wrote her family a note:

November 19, 2010

Dear Family of Jare Whitmore,

My name is Kim Clark and I am honored to be able to present this to you on behalf of my friend, Jare Whitmore.

The boxes here contain genuine kisses inside from Jare to you.

I collected them from her on Thursday, November 18th at approximately 4:30pm. I came to visit her and I shared my story with her.

Nearly 12 years ago my younger brother was losing his battle with a malignant brain tumor (he was 29).

Although we were facing the inevitable, I thought of a way of keeping a part of him here with me until we are reunited later in Heaven.

I came over prepared with a bag full of little boxes one night while we were over at his house watching a movie. I asked him if he would blow some kisses in the bag (I held it open). Without saying a word he blew kisses and I caught them.

Two nights later Sean passed away. The night he died I kept myself busy by putting the boxes together for everyone in our family.

I presented them at his funeral.

It's wonderful to always have a kiss from him, whenever I want and to share them with the people I love & the people he loves.

In June 2008 I was able to do the same (giving boxes of kisses) to the family of a friend,

Lori Ann Reid, she had Sarcoma the entire time I worked with her (all 4 years).

I know it hurts not having Jare here with us, but you should know that the box you hold are genuine....kisses from Jare; they are there for you whenever you want one.

I am very sorry for your loss but I look forward to sharing eternity with Jare some day.

Sincerely,
Kim Clark

I gave my mom the bag of wrapped kisses before we left on our trip. She brought the bag to church and gave it to a mutual friend (Francine) who delivered it to her husband. He sent word the boxes were a wonderful gift, and everybody was touched.

I love how God inspired me with the idea. It has given me a wonderful feeling, sharing this with other families. To be able to give them something so precious at a time of such great loss.

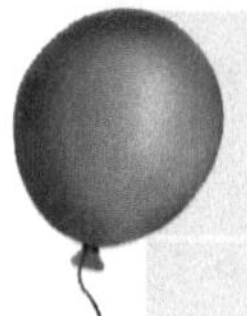

Remembering a special lady,
Jare Whitmore, who lost her battle
with cancer Nov. 23, 2010

Conclusion 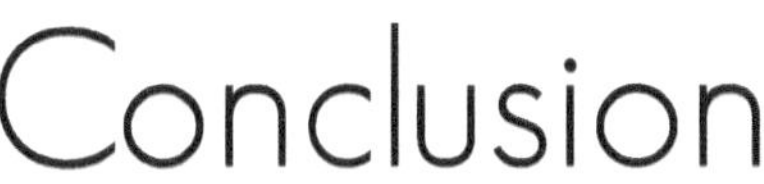

Kim – I'm happy to report after 2 ½ years I remain in remission.

I have regular scans as well as blood work. I will continue to see my Oncologist over the next 10 years, possibly longer.

Chemotherapy treatments have thrown me into menopause and also caused (Ok, helped) me gain a few pounds; radiation therapy has damaged my thyroid, but otherwise my health is good, thanks to God.

I knew one day I would go through menopause, I just never planned on going through it with my mother.

My hair grew back just as curly but very dense. I have a ton of hair!

I think there needs to be commercials on TV and TV shows with bald woman.

My nephew Sean – He is a happy, handsome 13 year old and lives with his mom, step dad and sister.

My parents celebrated their 50th wedding anniversary Nov. 13, 2010; surround by family and their closest friends at a wonderful gala held at the Hyatt Regency on the Bay in Sarasota. I'm happy and blessed to have been able to help bring this once in a lifetime occasion together for them. Thank you Aundria.

Losing someone I love so much, someone so close has been the hardest thing for me to live with. I never thought of going through life without him (my brother, Sean). I fight with the emotions of it all the time, but I found one way of dealing with it better....and when I think of the feelings of my loss in this way.....I do deal with it better. You see, God is the great planner, the great provider He created the heavens and the earth and everything in them and He gives us life. Once we have lived our life, we die and (Christians/Believers) are immediately "in the twinkling of an eye" we are in His presence. So, I couldn't think of a better way He would give us (Christians/Believers) our first day in eternity by nothing less than the greatest welcome we could imagine: by seeing the faces of those we love and have missed most greeting us at eternity's door.

Maybe all of us have to have someone close leave before us because it would be a pretty boring, maybe even confusing, way to arrive in eternity. Ok I'm here! But I don't know anyone no, it can't be that way. Every party we attend has people we know (hopefully) and like (hopefully), right? Would eternity start off with anything less?

You see, I'm looking forward to spending eternity with my brother and the rest of the family and my dear friends, those who died before and after his death and my own.

God must get excited about all these reunions. How great they must all be. I know how excited I was, planning my surprise visit to Florida. Eternity has to start off in some awesome way, don't you think? Well, that's what I believe.

Keep looking up!

Now let's hear your story.

E-mail me at: keeplookingupbook@comcast.net

or visit: www.keeplookingupbook.com

Author's Non-Profit Picks:

All Faiths Food Bank
8171 Blaikie Ct.
Sarasota, FL 34240
941-379-6333

The Leukemia & Lymphoma Society
Suncoast Chapter
3507 East Frontage Rd.
Tampa, FL 33607
(813) 963-6461
1-800-436-6889

Author's Local Business Picks

A Better Place Dance & Fitness Studio
2530 Bobcat Village Center Road
Port Charlotte, FL 34288
(941) 429-6700

Abracadabra Hair Studio
4183 Tamiami Trail S.
Venice, FL 34293
(941) 497-6988

Dr. Pascal Bordy
13815 Tamiami Trail
North Port, FL 34287
(941) 876-3597

Buffalo Wings & Rings
1081 W. Price Blvd.
North Port, FL 34288
(941) 257-2100

Cozy Caps available at
Murdock Baptist Church
Ask for Annette Hurley
941-627-6352

Dutch Valley Restaurant
6721 S. Tamiami Trail
Sarasota, FL 34231-4808
(941) 924-1770
Open Daily 7am-9am

Face 2 Face Ta2
Permanent Make Up
North Port, FL
(941) 426-3190 & (941) 650-8040
www.face2faceta2.com
face2faceta2@comcast.net

Florida Cancer Specialists
836 Sunset Lake Blvd., #101
Venice, FL
(941) 408-0500

Masterpiece Custom Homes
4535 West Price Boulevard
North Port, FL 34286
(941) 429-5355

North Port Taekwondo
14906 Tamiami Trail, Suite E
North Port, FL 34287
Phone: (941) 426-7484

Olde World Restaurant
14415 S. Tamiami Trail
North Port, FL 34287
(941) 426-1155

P-Nail Spa
1171 S. Toledo Blade Blvd.
North Port, FL 34288
(941) 426-9848

South Biscayne Baptist Church
13000 Tamiami Trail
North Port, FL 34287
(941) 426-3817